48 LAWS OF MENTAL POWER

Overcoming Trauma and Building Mental Strength

Victor O. Carl

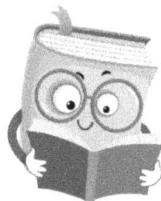

48LAWSOFLIFE
Making your life Better

Printed in the United States of America.

For more information, or to book an event, contact :
(Email & Website)
http://www.48lol.com
mail to : info@48lol.com

Book design by Joseph Campbell
Cover design by C.J (*D reinforced*)

ISBN – Ebook : 978-1-965849-06-4
ISBN - Paperback : 978-1-965849-07-1
ISBN - Hardcover : 978-1-965849-08-8

First Edition : September 2024

CONTENTS

Victor O. Carl

Thank you so much for purchasing my book!

I'm beyond excited to have you as part of my reading community. Your support truly means the world to me.

If you could kindly take a moment to scan the QR code below and share your honest review on Amazon, it would mean so much.

For those reading the ebook version, please click the link:

Amazon Review Link

Your feedback is invaluable—it helps me improve as a writer and strengthens our community. I genuinely love hearing from you and deeply appreciate your thoughts!

Preface

Unleashing Your Mental Power

In a world where physical strength and financial success are often celebrated, the true source of power lies in a domain far more subtle yet infinitely more impactful: the mind. The battles we face are rarely won or lost in the outer world but in the quiet arena of our own thoughts. The greatest victories, whether personal or professional, begin with mastering the most potent tool at our disposal: our mental power.

The 48 Laws of Mental Power is not just a guide—it is a roadmap to harnessing the untapped potential within you. It's a journey into the depths of your mind, where resilience is built, confidence is cultivated, and clarity is achieved. Every law within these pages is a key designed to unlock a higher level of personal mastery, empowering you to thrive in a chaotic world.

We are bombarded daily with distractions, fears, and self-doubt. The modern world tests our mental endurance, pushing us to the edge. But what if I told you that within you lies the strength to not only survive but to rise above? What if the secret to overcoming adversity, shaping your reality, and commanding the respect and influence you desire isn't found in external achievements, but in mastering the art of thinking?

This book was crafted for the modern warrior—a person determined to conquer not just the world but their own limitations. Through these 48 laws, you'll learn how to sharpen your focus, break free from mental chains, and channel your mind's full potential. From cultivating self-awareness to building mental resilience, from turning obstacles into opportunities to finding clarity in chaos—each law is a powerful tool designed to elevate your life.

The ancient Greek philosopher Epictetus once said, "No man is free who is not master of himself." This truth resonates more today than ever before. In these pages, you will discover how to become the master of your own mind—no longer a prisoner to circumstances, fears, or the opinions of others. You will learn how to shift your internal narrative, gain control over your thoughts, and harness the limitless power within.

Whether you seek personal growth, leadership, or simply peace of mind, the **48 Laws of Mental Power** will equip you with the strategies to thrive in every aspect of life. So, prepare to embark on this journey of self-mastery. The power you've been searching for has been within you all along.

INTRODUCTION

The global prevalence of mental health disorders is staggering, painting a picture of a world grappling with a silent crisis. The World Health Organization estimates that nearly **1 billion people** worldwide live with a mental disorder, with **depression** being a leading cause of disability globally. The burden of mental illness is particularly heavy on young people, with **half of all mental health conditions** starting by age 14 and 75% by age 24.

Anxiety disorders affect an estimated 284 million people globally, making them the most common mental health condition. Depression affects approximately 280 million people, with women being disproportionately affected. The global suicide rate is alarming, with one death every 40 seconds.[5] In 2020, over 700,000 people died by suicide, highlighting the urgent need for improved mental health care and suicide prevention efforts.

These numbers represent a global crisis that demands attention and action. The human cost of mental illness is immeasurable, affecting individuals, families, and communities worldwide. The economic burden is also significant, with mental health conditions costing the global economy an estimated US$ 1 trillion each year in lost productivity.

It is crucial to recognize that mental health is not a luxury but a fundamental human right. We must prioritize mental health care and invest in prevention and treatment efforts to address this global crisis. By breaking the silence and stigma surrounding mental illness, we can create a world where everyone has the opportunity to live a fulfilling and mentally healthy life.

Global Rise of Anxiety and Depression (1990-2025)

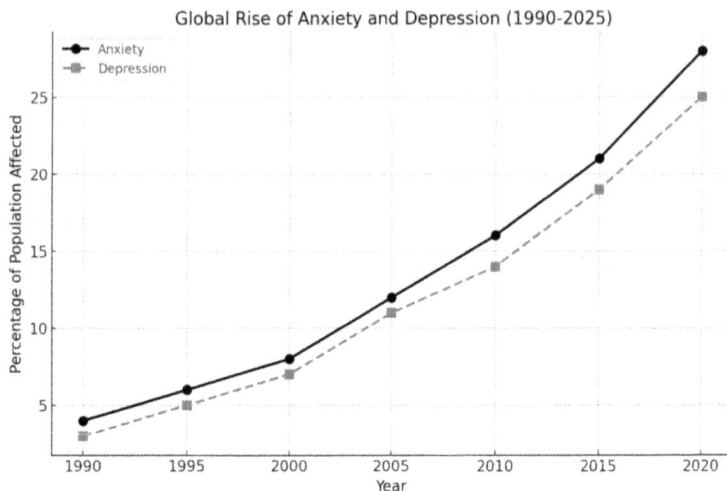

This graph illustrates the global rise of anxiety and depression from 1990 to 2025. The data shows a steady increase in the percentage of the population affected by both conditions.

These numbers are more than just statistics; they represent real people struggling in silence, their cries for help drowned out by the noise of everyday life. We're failing them, and we're failing ourselves.

The Silent Killer: Mental Health

While we obsess over visible threats like daibetes and cancer, we often neglect the silent killer that's claiming lives at an alarming rate: mental health disorders. Depression, anxiety, and the lingering effects of trauma are pervasive, affecting millions around the globe.

Here are some statistics on global mental health prevalence, with a particular focus on suicide rates:

- **Depression**: The World Health Organization estimates that over 264 million people worldwide suffer from depression, making it one of the leading causes of disability. It is more common in women than in men.

- **Anxiety**: Anxiety disorders affect an estimated 284 million people globally, also making it a major contributor to disability.
- **Suicide**: Approximately 703,000 people die by suicide each year, which equates to one death every 40 seconds. It is the fourth leading cause of death among 15-29-year-olds.
- **Global Burden**: Mental health conditions account for a significant portion of the global burden of disease. It is estimated that they contribute to 14% of all years lived with disability (YLDs).

Global Prevalence of Depression and Anxiety explained in a bar chart

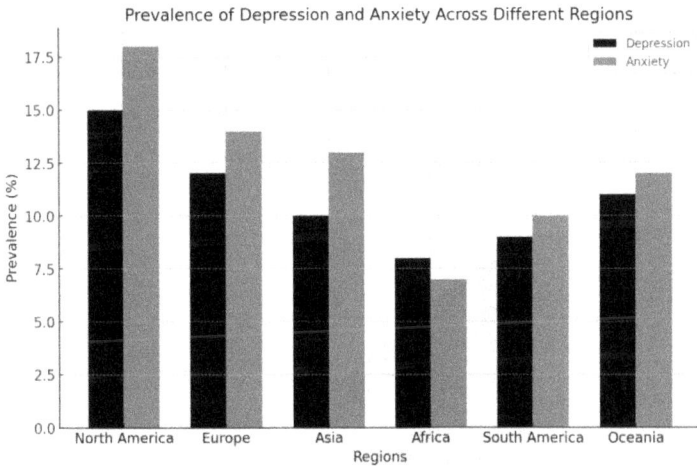

Prevalence of Depression and Anxiety Across Different Regions

Here is the bar chart comparing the prevalence of depression and anxiety across different regions of the world.

Suicide Rates by Age and Sex

Suicide Rates by Age Group and Gender (2000-2025)

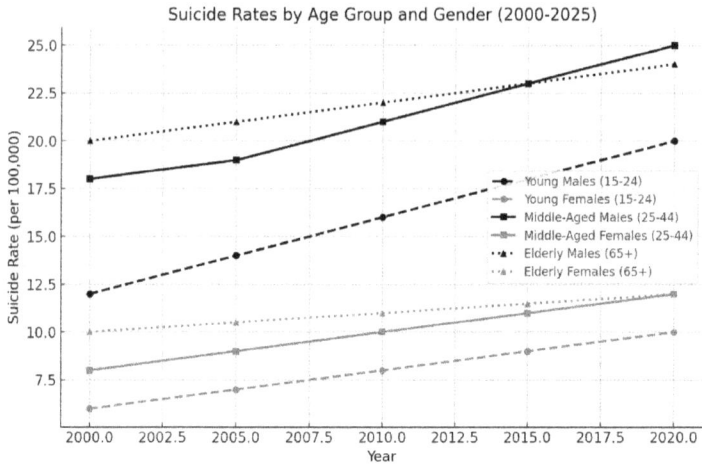

Legend:
- Young Males (15-24)
- Young Females (15-24)
- Middle-Aged Males (25-44)
- Middle-Aged Females (25-44)
- Elderly Males (65+)
- Elderly Females (65+)

Above is a line graph showing suicide rates by different age groups and genders from 2000 to 2025. The graph highlights the vulnerability of young people, with separate lines representing males and females from various age groups

Mental Health's Contribution to Global Disability

Global Disability Attributable to Health Conditions

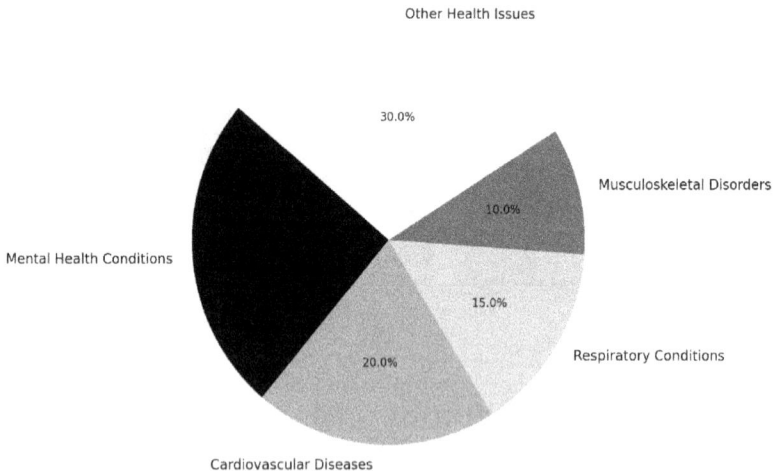

- Other Health Issues 30.0%
- Musculoskeletal Disorders 10.0%
- Respiratory Conditions 15.0%
- Cardiovascular Diseases 20.0%
- Mental Health Conditions

Here is the pie chart illustrating the percentage of global disability attributable to mental health conditions compared to other health issues.

Region	Prevalence of Depression (%)	Prevalence of Anxiety (%)	Suicide Rate (per 100,000)
Africa	4.4	3.4	11.2
Americas	5.0	7.3	10.3
South-East Asia	3.6	3.6	7.2
Europe	4.5	6.3	10.5
Eastern Mediterranean	3.9	4.0	5.9
Western Pacific	3.9	3.8	7.9

These statistics underscore the urgent need to address the global mental health crisis. It is a silent epidemic affecting millions of people across the world, impacting their lives, relationships, and overall well-being. The rising rates of anxiety, depression, and suicide, particularly among young people, highlight the critical need for increased awareness, accessible mental health services, and effective interventions to prevent and treat these conditions.

These numbers are a stark reminder that mental health is not a luxury but a necessity. Yet, it remains stigmatized, underfunded, and often misunderstood. We're quick to offer condolences when someone dies from a physical illness, but when someone takes their own life due to mental health struggles, we often whisper in hushed tones, unsure of what to say.

This silence is deadly. It perpetuates the myth that mental health is a personal failing, something to be ashamed of rather than addressed. It prevents people from seeking help, leaving them to battle their demons alone.

The 48 Laws of Mental Power: Your Savior

This book is a beacon of hope in the darkness. It's a guide to reclaiming your mental and emotional well-being, to building the resilience needed to navigate life's challenges. It's about understanding that mental health is not a fixed state but a dynamic process that requires constant attention and care.

Just as we prioritize physical health through exercise and nutrition, we must also prioritize our mental health through intentional practices and self-awareness. The 48 Laws of Mental Power offers a roadmap to that journey, providing you with the tools and strategies to cultivate a mind that is strong, resilient, and capable of overcoming any obstacle.

It's time to break the silence, to shed the stigma, and to embrace the power of mental well-being. Your journey to a happier, healthier, and more fulfilling life starts now.

This book is your lifeline. It's about equipping you with the tools to navigate life's complexities with strength, clarity, and purpose. It's about reclaiming your mental and emotional well-being, one law at a time.

Through practical steps, you'll learn to:

- Master your thoughts and emotions
- Overcome the lingering effects of trauma
- Build unshakeable resilience
- Cultivate inner peace and joy
- Unleash your full potential

Whether you're battling anxiety, wrestling with the demons of your past, or simply seeking to enhance your mental well-being, this book is your guide. It's time to break free from the limitations of your past, embrace your innate resilience, and step into a life of purpose, joy, and unwavering mental power.

Remember, the power to change your life lies within you. This book is the key to unlocking that power.

The 48 Laws of Mental Power

Law 1: Embrace Reality

- Denial is a prison; freedom begins with acceptance; *The Body Keeps the Score* teaches us that trauma is stored in the body and mind. Embracing reality means acknowledging the trauma and its effects rather than denying or avoiding it. Only by confronting the truth can healing begin.

Law 2: Allow Yourself to Feel

- Your emotions are your compass—don't ignore their direction; Trauma disrupts the connection between mind and body, often leading to emotional numbness. Allowing yourself to feel is about reconnecting with your emotions, no matter how painful, so that you can process and release them.

Law 3: Seek the Guide

- The right mentor can turn darkness into light; Just as Van der Kolk emphasizes the importance of professional help, this law encourages seeking out therapists or counselors who can help you navigate the complexities of trauma, providing the tools needed for recovery.

Law 4: Build Your Fortress

- A strong support system is your shield against the storm; A strong support system is vital. Surround yourself with people who understand and support your healing process, creating a safe space where you can be vulnerable and grow stronger.

Law 5: Be Your Own Best Friend

- Show yourself the kindness you've always deserved; Trauma often breeds self-criticism. This law urges you to counteract that by practicing self-compassion, treating yourself with the kindness and understanding that you would offer to a dear friend.

Law 6: Conquer in Small Steps

- Giant leaps are overrated; true progress is gradual; Recovery isn't a sprint; it's a marathon. By setting small, achievable goals, you can avoid feeling overwhelmed and build momentum, reinforcing your progress one step at a time.

Law 7: Control the Controllables

- Focus your energy where it matters most; In the aftermath of trauma, it's easy to feel powerless. This law focuses on regaining a sense of control by concentrating on what you can influence—your actions, responses, and choices.

Law 8: Find Your Escape

- Healthy outlets are the keys to maintaining sanity; Healthy coping mechanisms, such as exercise, journaling, or creative outlets, allow you to process emotions and reduce stress, offering a productive escape from the intensity of your feelings.

Law 9: Stay Present

- The past is a shadow; the future, a mirage. Only the present is real; Trauma often keeps us stuck in the past or anxious about the future. Mindfulness practices help anchor you in the present moment, reducing the grip of traumatic memories and future worries.

Law 10: Create Rituals

- Routines are the anchors that keep you grounded;
Routines provide stability in the chaotic aftermath of
trauma. Establishing daily rituals—like morning coffee,
exercise, or meditation—can ground you and create a
sense of normalcy.

Law 11: Prioritize Rest

- Your mind cannot heal without proper rest; Trauma
affects the body's ability to rest and recover. Prioritizing
sleep is essential, as it allows your body and mind to heal
and regenerate, helping to alleviate the symptoms of
trauma.

Law 12: Feed the Mind, Feed the Body

- What nourishes you sustains you—inside and out;
Nutrition plays a crucial role in mental health. A balanced
diet can improve mood, increase energy levels, and help
stabilize emotions, which is critical in the healing process.

Law 13: Move to Heal

- Physical movement is a balm for a weary mind; Physical
activity is a powerful way to release the stress and
tension stored in the body due to trauma. Exercise helps
reconnect the mind and body, promoting overall well-
being.

Law 14: Resist the False Friends

- Substance abuse promises relief but delivers destruction;
Substances like alcohol and drugs may seem like an easy
way to numb the pain, but they ultimately exacerbate the
problem. True healing requires confronting trauma, not
avoiding it.

Law 15: Cultivate Gratitude

- Gratitude is the antidote to despair; Practicing gratitude
shifts your focus from what's wrong to what's right. This

simple act can transform your perspective, reducing stress and increasing resilience.

Law 16: Know Your Triggers

- Awareness is the first line of defense against the past; Understanding what triggers your trauma responses is crucial. By identifying these triggers, you can prepare for them and develop strategies to manage them effectively.

Law 17: Reframe Your Thoughts

- Your thoughts are the architects of your reality; Negative thought patterns are common in trauma survivors. Reframing these thoughts—turning "I'm broken" into "I'm healing"—can change your mindset and empower your recovery.

Law 18: Release Resentment

- Forgiveness is the ultimate act of self-liberation; Holding onto anger and resentment can poison your spirit. Forgiveness isn't about excusing what happened; it's about freeing yourself from the burden of bitterness.

Law 19: Establish Your Boundaries

- Boundaries are the lines that protect your peace; Trauma often leaves us vulnerable to further harm. Setting clear boundaries is a way of protecting your peace and ensuring that you only allow supportive, positive influences into your life.

Law 20: Reconnect with the Earth

- Nature is a healer that asks nothing in return; Nature has a profound ability to heal. Spending time outdoors can calm your nervous system, reduce stress, and help you feel more connected and grounded.

Law 21: Rediscover Joy

- Hobbies are the seeds of joy that grow in the heart; Hobbies and activities that bring you joy are essential for healing. They remind you that life is about more than just surviving—it's about finding moments of happiness and fulfillment.

Law 22: Arm Yourself with Knowledge

- Knowledge turns fear into understanding; Understanding the science of trauma, as explained in *The Body Keeps the Score*, empowers you to take control of your healing. Knowledge is a powerful tool in overcoming the effects of trauma.

Law 23: Express Without Words

- Creativity is the voice that speaks when words fail; Sometimes, words are not enough to express the depth of your emotions. Creative outlets like art, music, or dance can help you process and release feelings that are difficult to verbalize.

Law 24: Test Your Limits

- Strength is found in the stretch beyond comfort; Healing involves growth, and growth often happens when you push beyond your comfort zone. Gradually challenging yourself can help rebuild your confidence and resilience.

Law 25: Trust the Process

- Patience is the quiet power that sustains the journey; Healing from trauma is a journey with ups and downs. Patience is key—trust that each step, no matter how small, is moving you toward recovery.

Law 26: Stay Engaged

- Isolation is the enemy; connection is the cure. Trauma often leads to isolation, but staying connected with others is crucial. Engaging with supportive communities or loved ones can provide the connection needed to heal.

Law 27: Learn to Say No

- Protect your energy by mastering the art of refusal; Protecting your mental health means setting boundaries and learning to say no to demands that drain you or cause stress. Prioritize your well-being over pleasing others.

Law 28: Celebrate the Small Wins

- Progress is built on the foundation of small victories; Every step forward, no matter how small, is a victory. Recognizing and celebrating these achievements helps build momentum and reinforces your progress.

Law 29: Embrace Your Unique Path

- Comparisons are thieves; your journey is yours alone. Everyone's healing journey is different. Avoid comparing yourself to others and focus on your own progress, recognizing that your path is uniquely yours.

Law 30: Master the Breath

- Breath control is the key to controlling the mind; Breathing exercises can calm your mind and body, reducing anxiety and stress. Mastering the breath is a powerful tool in managing trauma responses.

Law 31: Write Your Story

- The pen is mightier when used to understand oneself; Journaling or writing your experiences can be a therapeutic way to process trauma. It allows you to externalize your thoughts and gain clarity on your emotions.

Law 32: Recognize Your Strength

- Your past victories are proof of your resilience; Trauma may make you feel weak, but surviving it is a testament to your strength. Recognize and honor the resilience that has brought you this far.

Law 33: Rebuild Trust Slowly

- Trust is a fragile thing, but it can be mended; Trust is often shattered by trauma. Rebuilding it—both in yourself and in others—takes time, but it's essential for restoring healthy relationships.

Law 34: Eliminate the Toxic

- Remove the poison to allow the healing; Toxic relationships or environments can hinder your recovery. Removing these influences is crucial to creating a safe space for healing.

Law 35: Learn the Science

- Understanding trauma unlocks the door to recovery; Understanding the physiological and psychological effects of trauma can help demystify your experiences and empower your recovery process.

Law 36: Give Back to Heal

- In serving others, you find your own salvation; Helping others who are struggling can provide a sense of purpose and fulfillment, aiding in your own healing journey.

Law 37: Turn Setbacks into Lessons

- Every fall is a step toward mastery; Setbacks are a natural part of the healing process. Rather than seeing them as failures, view them as opportunities to learn and grow stronger.

Law 38: Stay Open to New Beginnings

- The unknown holds the keys to your future; Trauma can close you off to new experiences. Staying open to new opportunities and possibilities can lead to unexpected growth and joy.

Law 39: Build Resilience from Adversity

- The strongest steel is forged in the hottest fire; Adversity builds resilience. Each challenge you overcome makes you stronger, preparing you for whatever lies ahead.

Law 40: Live in the Now

- The present moment is the only reality you truly control; The present moment is where healing occurs. Focus on the here and now to reduce anxiety and connect with your inner peace.

Law 41: Find Meaning in Pain

- Even suffering has something to teach; Finding meaning in your trauma can transform your pain into a source of strength and purpose, helping you to move forward.

Law 42: Realign Your Priorities

- Trauma reshapes you; let it guide you to what truly matters; Trauma often forces a reassessment of what truly matters. Use this as an opportunity to realign your life with your core values and goals.

Law 43: Seek Inner Peace

- Peace is not found; it is cultivated. Inner peace doesn't mean the absence of conflict, but the ability to maintain calm amidst life's challenges. Cultivate practices that nurture this peace within you.

Law 44: Be Consistent in Your Practices

- Consistency is the mother of lasting change; Consistency in your healing practices—whether it's therapy, mindfulness, or self-care—leads to sustained progress and deeper recovery.

Law 45: Honor Your Progress

- Every step forward deserves recognition; Acknowledge how far you've come. Reflecting on your progress reinforces your resilience and motivates you to keep moving forward.

Law 46: Rediscover Who You Are

- Trauma can obscure, but it can also reveal your true self; Trauma can obscure your sense of self. Take time to reconnect with your identity, passions, and what makes you unique.

Law 47: Embrace the Journey

- Healing is a path, not a destination; Healing is not a destination but a continuous journey. Embrace the process, with all its ups and downs, as part of your growth.

Law 48: Believe in Your Power

- You are stronger than you know; resilience is your birthright; Your ability to heal is greater than you realize. Trust in your inner strength and resilience—you have the power to overcome and thrive.

Law 1:

EMBRACE REALITY

"We cannot change anything until we accept it. Condemnation does not liberate, it oppresses."
Carl Jung

During World War II, Viktor Frankl, an Austrian psychiatrist, found himself imprisoned in the most harrowing of conditions—Nazi concentration camps, including Auschwitz. Stripped of his family, his freedom, and his identity, Frankl was subjected to unimaginable suffering. Amidst the brutality, Frankl made a pivotal realization: while he could not control the horrors around him, he could control his response to them. He embraced the brutal reality of his situation, not as a passive acceptance, but as an active choice to find meaning in his suffering. This approach enabled him to endure the unendurable and later inspired his development of logotherapy, a form of psychotherapy centered on finding meaning even in the darkest of circumstances.

Understanding the 1st Law:
Viktor Frankl's experience teaches us that the foundation of mental resilience is the ability to embrace reality as it is, not as we wish it to be. Trauma and stress disrupt the balance between the rational and emotional parts of the brain, often pushing us into states of hyperarousal (where we feel overwhelmed and reactive)

or hyperarousal (where we feel numb and disconnected). These states take us outside our "window of tolerance," the range in which we function optimally and maintain emotional stability.

When we are outside this window, our mind and body are in disarray. We become reactive, disorganized, and unable to learn from our experiences because our internal alarms are either blaring or completely shut down. The key to recovery, as Frankl discovered, lies in restoring balance—bringing the emotional brain back to its role as a quiet background presence that supports our daily life without overwhelming it.

Practical Steps To Achieving the 1st Law of Mental Power:

Develop Self-Awareness: The first step in embracing reality is becoming aware of your internal state—your emotions, bodily sensations, and the thoughts that arise within you. This process, known as interoception, involves "looking inside" and noticing what is happening within.

Mindfulness Practices: By engaging in mindfulness, you can observe your internal experiences without judgment. This practice helps you separate your identity from your immediate reactions, allowing you to regain control over your responses to stress and trauma.

Regulate Your Emotions: Awareness alone is not enough; you must also learn to regulate your emotions. Emotional regulation is critical in managing trauma responses and restoring internal balance.

Breathing Techniques: Simple practices like deep, slow breathing can calm your nervous system, reducing the intensity of hyperarousal. By focusing on your breath, you engage the parasympathetic nervous system, which acts as a brake on your fight-or-flight responses, helping you stay grounded even when facing distressing memories.

Movement and Relaxation: Incorporating physical activities like yoga or tai chi can reduce PTSD symptoms and help regulate your body's response to stress. By moving deliberately and focusing on your body's sensations, you retrain your mind to remain calm and present.

Integrate the Emotional and Rational Brains: True recovery involves not just calming the emotional brain but also re-engaging the rational brain. This integration allows you to approach life with flexibility, creativity, and confidence, rather than being rigid or reactive.

Limbic System Therapy: This approach involves "repairing" the emotional brain so it can resume its normal role—monitoring your environment and responding appropriately without overwhelming your rational brain. Techniques like mindfulness, neurofeedback, and somatic experiencing help restore this balance, making you less likely to be hijacked by your emotions.

Mind-Body Practices: Engage in practices like martial arts, rhythmic drumming, or meditation, which not only engage the body but also calm the mind, allowing your emotional brain to function as a supportive, rather than disruptive, presence.

Stay in the Present Moment: Trauma often traps you in the past or makes you anxious about the future. By staying present, you reclaim your power over your life. The more you can ground yourself in the here and now, the more you reduce the influence of traumatic memories.

Mindfulness and Body Awareness: Regularly practice mindfulness to stay connected to the present. Focus on your breathing, body sensations, and the simple experiences of daily life. This helps you stay within your window of tolerance, where you can think clearly and respond to life's challenges with resilience.

Embracing reality, as Viktor Frankl exemplified, is about restoring balance within yourself by reconnecting your emotional and rational brains. Through self-awareness, emotional regulation, and mindfulness, you can regain control over how you respond to the world. This process is the foundation of mental resilience, enabling you to face life's challenges with clarity, strength, and an empowered sense of self. Just as Frankl found meaning in his suffering, you too can find strength in embracing the reality of your experiences, no matter how difficult they may be.

Law 2

ALLOW YOURSELF TO FEEL

"You can't heal what you don't feel."— *Anonymous*

Eleanor Roosevelt is often remembered as one of the most influential First Ladies in American history. But before she became a beacon of strength and compassion, Eleanor's life was marked by deep personal struggles. Born into a wealthy family, she endured a childhood filled with sorrow. By the age of ten, Eleanor had lost both of her parents—her mother to diphtheria and her father, whom she adored, to alcoholism and suicide. These early tragedies left her feeling abandoned and insecure, casting a long shadow over her formative years.

As Eleanor grew older, her struggles did not dissipate. Her marriage to Franklin D. Roosevelt was marred by betrayal when she discovered his affair with her social secretary, Lucy Mercer. This revelation devastated her, shaking the foundation of her personal life. Yet, instead of succumbing to bitterness or closing herself off from the world, Eleanor chose a different path—one of emotional honesty and resilience.

Eleanor realized that the only way to truly heal and find her voice was to confront her emotions head-on. She allowed herself to feel the full spectrum of her pain, disappointment, and fear. Rather than suppressing these feelings, she embraced them, understanding that they were a natural response to her experiences. This process of emotional acceptance became a turning point in her life.

By allowing herself to feel, Eleanor began to transform her pain into purpose. She channeled her emotional depth into her work, advocating for human rights, social justice, and the empowerment of women. Her ability to connect with people from all walks of life, empathize with their struggles, and fight for their rights stemmed from her journey through emotional hardship. Eleanor's legacy as a compassionate leader was built on the foundation of her willingness to feel deeply and authentically.

Her story illustrates the second law of mental power: Allow Yourself to Feel. It is through the full acknowledgment and acceptance of our emotions—no matter how painful—that we can truly heal, grow, and find strength.

Understanding the 2nd Law:

In the quest for mental resilience, one of the most important steps is to allow yourself to fully experience your emotions. Trauma and stress often lead people to suppress or avoid their feelings, believing that this will protect them from further pain. However, this avoidance only exacerbates the problem, trapping you in a cycle of unprocessed emotions that can manifest in harmful ways—whether through anxiety, depression, or even physical illness.

Avoiding your emotions can keep you in a state of hyperarousal, where you are constantly on edge, anxious, and reactive, or hyperarousal, where you feel numb, detached, and unable to engage with life. These states are symptomatic of a brain that is disconnected from its emotional core—a state that *The Body Keeps the Score* refers to as the disconnection between the rational and emotional brains. To heal, you must reconnect these parts of your mind, allowing yourself to feel and process your emotions fully.

Practical Steps To Achieving the 2nd Law of Mental Power:

Acknowledge Your Emotions: The first step in allowing yourself to feel is acknowledging that your emotions are valid and real. Just as Eleanor Roosevelt did, recognize that your feelings—whether they be anger, sadness, or fear—are natural responses to your life experiences. Acknowledging them is the first step toward healing.

Mindful Observation: Start by practicing mindfulness, which involves observing your emotions without judgment. Notice where these emotions manifest in your body. Do you feel a tightness in your chest, a knot in your stomach, or a lump in your throat? By identifying these physical sensations, you begin to process your emotions more effectively.

Practice Emotional Regulation: After acknowledging your emotions, the next step is to regulate them. Emotional regulation doesn't mean suppressing your feelings; it means managing them in a way that allows you to stay balanced and in control.

Breathing Techniques: One of the most effective ways to regulate your emotions is through deep breathing. When you find yourself overwhelmed, take a few deep, slow breaths. Focus on the sensation of air entering and leaving your lungs. This simple act can calm your nervous system, reducing the intensity of your emotions and helping you return to a state of equilibrium.

Movement and Relaxation: Incorporating physical activities like yoga, tai chi, or mindful walking into your routine can also help regulate your emotions. These practices encourage the release of physical tension, which often accompanies strong emotions, allowing you to process your feelings more effectively.

Label Your Emotions: Naming your emotions is a powerful way to take control of them. When you give your feelings a name—whether it's anxiety, sadness, or anger—you help your brain process these emotions more clearly.

Self-Reflection: Take time to reflect on what you're feeling and why. For instance, if you're feeling anxious, identify the physical sensation, like a racing heart or sweating palms, and label it as anxiety. This practice not only helps you understand your emotions better but also diminishes their intensity.

Create a Safe Space to Feel: It's crucial to create an environment where you feel safe to explore your emotions. This might be a physical space, like a quiet room, or a mental space, such as a meditation practice, where you can confront your feelings without fear.

Journaling: Writing about your emotions can be an incredibly effective way to process them. By putting your feelings into words, you create a narrative that helps you make sense of your emotions and reduces their power over you.

Understand the Transience of Emotions: Emotions are not permanent; they ebb and flow like waves. Understanding that your feelings are temporary can help you avoid being overwhelmed by them.

Mindfulness Practice: Regular mindfulness practice can help you stay connected to the present moment. Focus on the transient nature of your emotions, noticing how they rise and fall. This awareness can keep you grounded and prevent you from being swept away by intense feelings.

Allowing yourself to feel is an essential part of building mental resilience. By acknowledging, regulating, and processing your emotions, you take control of your inner world. This law teaches that emotions are not to be feared but are integral to your healing journey. Eleanor Roosevelt's transformation from a woman burdened by sorrow to a leader of immense compassion and strength was rooted in her willingness to feel deeply. By embracing your emotions, you too can unlock your inner power and transform your pain into purpose.

The 48 Laws of Mental Power

Law 3

"A mentor is someone who allows you to see the hope inside yourself."— Oprah Winfrey

When navigating the complexities of trauma, abuse, or significant emotional distress, the guidance of a competent therapist can be invaluable. The process of healing is intricate, requiring a deep understanding of how trauma affects the mind and body. Therefore, choosing the right therapist is a critical step in your journey toward recovery and mental resilience.

Competent trauma therapists undergo extensive training to understand the profound impact of trauma, abuse, and neglect on individuals. This training equips them with the necessary skills to stabilize and calm their patients, help them process and integrate traumatic memories, and ultimately reconnect them with others in a meaningful way. The effectiveness of therapy often hinges on the therapist's ability to master a variety of techniques, adapt them to the specific needs of the patient, and foster a safe, trusting environment.

Research supports the importance of therapeutic competence in trauma treatment. A study published in the *Journal of Traumatic Stress* highlights that effective trauma therapy often involves a combination of approaches tailored to the individual's needs. Techniques such as Eye Movement Desensitization and

Reprocessing (EMDR), Cognitive Behavioral Therapy (CBT), and somatic therapies have all shown efficacy in treating trauma, but their success largely depends on the therapist's expertise and flexibility in applying them.

How to Choose the Right Therapist:

Assess the Therapist's Training and Experience: It is crucial to choose a therapist who has received specialized training in trauma therapy. A well-trained therapist should have a thorough understanding of the various methods available for treating trauma and should be able to explain these approaches to you. It's perfectly reasonable to ask potential therapists about their training, where they acquired their skills, and whether they have personally benefited from the therapies they practice.

Key Questions to Ask: What specific training have you received in trauma therapy? Which therapeutic approaches do you use, and why? Have you found these approaches personally beneficial in your practice?

Evaluate the Therapist's Openness and Flexibility: There is no single "treatment of choice" for trauma, and the best therapists recognize this. A competent therapist will be open to exploring different therapeutic options and willing to adapt their approach based on what works best for you. Be wary of therapists who insist that their method is the only answer to your problems; such rigidity may indicate an ideological rather than a patient-centered approach.

Collaboration in Therapy: Effective therapy is a collaborative process. A good therapist will not only apply their expertise but also remain open to learning from you, adapting their methods to better suit your unique needs and experiences.

Ensure a Sense of Safety and Comfort: The therapeutic relationship is built on trust and safety. You should feel comfortable with your therapist, sensing that they are genuinely interested in understanding you as an individual, not just as a set of symptoms. Feeling safe with your therapist is essential for you to confront your fears and anxieties. A therapist who is stern, judgmental, or harsh is unlikely to create the supportive environment necessary for healing.

Therapeutic Alliance: Research published in the *Journal of Counseling Psychology* emphasizes that the therapeutic alliance— the collaborative and trusting relationship between therapist and patient—is one of the most significant predictors of successful therapy outcomes. If you feel safe and understood by your therapist, you are more likely to engage fully in the therapeutic process and achieve positive results.

Consider Personal Fit and Connection: Beyond credentials and techniques, the personal connection you feel with your therapist plays a crucial role in your healing journey. Your therapist must be not only competent but also capable of making you feel heard, respected, and valued as a person. This connection fosters a sense of trust that allows you to open up and engage deeply with the therapeutic process.

Personal Connection: Does your therapist seem comfortable in their skin? Do they make you feel at ease during sessions? These factors contribute to a positive therapeutic environment where you can explore and heal from your trauma.

Explore Alternative Therapies and Supports: In some cases, traditional talk therapy might not be sufficient or may not feel like the right fit for you. Alternative therapies, such as animal-assisted therapy, art therapy, or movement-based practices like yoga or tai chi, can offer additional avenues for healing. For example, equine therapy, where patients interact with horses, is particularly effective for trauma survivors who struggle to feel safe with other people.

Case Example: In a therapeutic setting, a young girl named Jennifer found solace and a sense of responsibility through caring for a horse. This bond helped her feel safe enough to begin relating to the staff at her treatment center, ultimately leading to her academic and personal success.

Choosing the right therapist is a critical component of seeking the guidance you need on your journey toward mental resilience. A competent therapist not only brings expertise and specialized training to the table but also creates a safe, trusting environment where you can explore your emotions and experiences. Remember that therapy is a collaborative process; your therapist should be open to adapting their methods to meet your unique needs and exploring various treatment options that best support your healing. By carefully selecting a therapist who fits these criteria, you can ensure that you are on the path to effective recovery and growth.

Law 4

BUILD YOUR FORTRESS - A SECURE BASE

"When we are no longer able to change a situation, we are challenged to change ourselves." Viktol Frankl.

The story of Nelson Mandela is a powerful testament to the concept of building a secure base—a principle at the heart of the fourth law of mental resilience, "Build Your Fortress." Mandela, who became a global symbol of resistance against oppression, found the strength to endure nearly three decades of imprisonment and ultimately lead his nation to freedom through the secure base he built both in his early life and during his years of struggle.

Nelson Mandela's Secure Base

Born in 1918 in the rural village of Mvezo, South Africa, Nelson Mandela grew up in the Thembu royal family. His early life was marked by a strong sense of tradition, community, and connection to his cultural roots. Mandela's father died when he was young, but he was taken in by Chief Jongintaba Dalindyebo, the acting regent of the Thembu people. This move provided Mandela with a secure base—a stable and nurturing environment where he could develop a sense of identity, purpose, and responsibility.

Chief Jongintaba and Mandela's other guardians instilled in him the values of leadership, justice, and duty. This upbringing gave Mandela the emotional and psychological resilience he would later draw upon during his long fight against apartheid. His secure base, grounded in the teachings of his elders and the traditions of his people, provided him with the inner strength to face the immense challenges that lay ahead.

The Role of a Secure Base During Mandela's Imprisonment

Mandela's 27 years of imprisonment on Robben Island were marked by extreme hardship. Cut off from the outside world, subjected to harsh conditions, and separated from his family, Mandela relied heavily on the secure base he had built within himself. The resilience he displayed during these years was not just a product of physical endurance but of a deeply rooted psychological stability that had been nurtured since childhood.

Even in the most isolating and dehumanizing conditions, Mandela maintained his sense of purpose. He stayed connected to his values, his vision for a free South Africa, and the relationships he had cultivated with his fellow prisoners. These connections became a new kind of secure base, helping him maintain his mental and emotional well-being. Mandela's ability to foster a sense of community even within the walls of a prison exemplifies the power of a secure base to provide strength and resilience in the face of adversity.

When he was finally released in 1990, Mandela emerged not as a broken man, but as a leader ready to guide his nation through a peaceful transition to democracy. The secure base he had built throughout his life enabled him to forgive his oppressors, advocate for reconciliation, and lead South Africa into a new era.

Achieving a Secure Base in Your Own Life

Nelson Mandela's life teaches us the immense power of a secure base—a foundation of emotional and psychological safety that allows us to explore, grow, and face challenges with resilience. To build your secure base, consider the following steps:

1. **Cultivate Meaningful Relationships**: Just as Mandela relied on his relationships with fellow prisoners and his memories of home, you can strengthen your resilience by nurturing relationships that provide emotional support and stability. These relationships should be based on mutual trust, respect, and understanding.

2. **Create a Safe Physical and Emotional Space**: Mandela's prison cell became a place of inner reflection and strength because he maintained his mental fortitude and emotional resilience. Similarly, you can create a haven in your life by cultivating environments where you feel secure and at peace. This could be a physical space, like your home, or an emotional space, like a supportive relationship.

3. **Practice Self-Regulation**: Mandela's ability to remain calm and composed under pressure was key to his survival and success. You can develop similar self-regulation skills through practices like mindfulness, meditation, or other techniques that help you manage stress and maintain emotional balance.

4. **Stay Connected to Your Values and Purpose**: Throughout his imprisonment, Mandela never lost sight of his goal of achieving freedom for his people. By staying connected to your core values and purpose, you can build a secure base that will guide you through difficult times.

5. **Seek Professional Guidance if Needed**: If past traumas or unresolved emotional issues are hindering your ability to feel secure, consider seeking help from a therapist or counselor. Professional guidance can help you address

these challenges and build a more secure foundation for your mental health.

The fourth law of mental resilience, "Build Your Fortress," underscores the importance of establishing a secure base in your life. Nelson Mandela's story exemplifies how a secure base, whether formed in childhood or cultivated in the harshest of circumstances, can provide the foundation for remarkable resilience and strength. By creating a secure base through meaningful relationships, safe spaces, self-regulation, and a strong connection to your values, you can build your inner fortress, enabling you to face life's challenges with the same resilience that Mandela displayed throughout his life.

Law 5

Be Your Own Best Friend

"You have been criticizing yourself for years, and it hasn't worked. Try approving of yourself and see what happens." Louise Hay

The fifth law of mental resilience, "Be Your Own Best Friend," speaks to the critical need for self-compassion in the journey toward mental strength and well-being. Trauma and adversity often breed self-criticism, making it difficult for individuals to treat themselves with the kindness they deserve. This law urges us to counteract self-criticism by practicing self-compassion and treating ourselves with the same understanding and kindness that we would offer to a dear friend.

The Power of Self-Compassion

Self-compassion is a fundamental aspect of mental resilience. It involves recognizing our suffering, responding to it with kindness and understanding, and treating ourselves with the care we would offer others in a similar situation. This practice is essential because, as human beings, we are wired for connection and kindness. As Jerome Kagan, a distinguished professor of child psychology, observed, for every act of cruelty in the world, there are countless acts of kindness and connection. This inclination toward benevolence is a true feature of our species, one that we must extend toward ourselves, especially in times of difficulty.

The Dalai Lama's teachings often emphasize the importance of self-compassion, aligning with Kagan's observation. He suggests that when we show kindness to ourselves, we create a foundation of inner peace and stability that enables us to extend kindness to others. This idea is closely tied to mental health, as feeling safe and secure in our own minds is essential for establishing meaningful connections with others and leading a satisfying life.

A powerful example of self-compassion in action can be found in the life of Maya Angelou, the renowned poet, author, and civil rights activist. Angelou's early life was marked by significant trauma, including sexual abuse and abandonment. These experiences could have easily led her down a path of self-criticism and despair. Instead, Angelou learned to be her own best friend, cultivating a deep sense of self-compassion that allowed her to overcome her past and achieve greatness.

After her traumatic childhood, Angelou spent years as a mute, unable to speak due to the psychological impact of her experiences. During this period, she turned to books and literature, which became her sanctuary. Through reading, she found voices of strength and wisdom that helped her reconnect with her own voice. This self-compassionate approach—allowing herself the time and space to heal and rediscover her identity—eventually led her to become one of the most powerful literary voices of the 20th century.

Angelou's ability to show herself kindness and understanding in the face of profound trauma exemplifies the essence of this law. By being her own best friend, she not only healed her wounds but also transformed her pain into art that has inspired millions around the world.

Achieving This Law: A Personal Experience

In my own life, I have found that practicing self-compassion has been a crucial part of maintaining mental resilience. A few years ago, I was going through a particularly challenging time. The pressure to meet expectations, both personal and professional, had become overwhelming, and I found myself trapped in a cycle of self-criticism and doubt.

During this period, I remembered a piece of advice I had once read: "Talk to yourself as you would talk to someone you love." It was a simple idea, but it resonated deeply with me. I realized that I had been treating myself with far less kindness and understanding than I would offer to a friend in the same situation.

I began to practice self-compassion by consciously changing my inner dialogue. Instead of criticizing myself for every perceived failure, I started acknowledging my efforts and reminding myself that it was okay to struggle. I allowed myself to rest when needed, and I made time for activities that brought me joy and relaxation. Over time, this practice of being my own best friend helped me regain my sense of balance and perspective. I became more resilient, not because the challenges disappeared, but because I approached them from a place of self-compassion rather than self-criticism.

How to Practice Self-Compassion

Practicing self-compassion is a skill that can be developed over time. Here are some steps to help you embody this law in your own life:

1. **Mindful Awareness**: The first step in practicing self-compassion is to become aware of your inner dialogue. Notice when you are being self-critical or harsh with yourself. Mindfulness allows you to observe your thoughts without judgment and recognize when you need to offer yourself kindness.

2. **Self-Kindness**: When you catch yourself being self-critical, pause and ask yourself how you would speak to a dear friend in the same situation. Offer yourself words of encouragement and support. Remind yourself that it's okay to make mistakes and that you are deserving of love and kindness.

3. **Common Humanity**: Remember that everyone struggles and experiences failure. You are not alone in your suffering. Recognizing that others share similar experiences can help you feel more connected and less isolated in your difficulties.

4. **Forgiveness**: Allow yourself to forgive your past mistakes and shortcomings. Holding onto guilt and regret can prevent you from moving forward. Embrace the idea that you are a work in progress and that personal growth involves making mistakes and learning from them.

5. **Seek Support**: Sometimes, self-compassion requires reaching out for help. Whether it's talking to a trusted friend, family member, or therapist, seeking support when you're struggling is a powerful act of self-care.

The fifth law of mental resilience, "Be Your Own Best Friend," highlights the importance of self-compassion in building mental strength and well-being. Through the example of Maya Angelou and the teachings of thinkers like the Dalai Lama, we see how self-compassion can transform trauma and adversity into growth and resilience. By practicing self-compassion—through mindful awareness, self-kindness, embracing common humanity, forgiving ourselves, and seeking support—we can cultivate a deep inner resilience that allows us to navigate life's challenges with grace and strength. In doing so, we become not only our own best friends but also more compassionate and understanding toward others.

Law 6

Conquer in Small Steps

"The man who moves a mountain begins by carrying away small stones." Confucius

The sixth law of mental resilience, "Conquer in Small Steps," emphasizes the importance of gradual, incremental progress over the allure of giant leaps. Recovery and personal growth are not races to be won in one dramatic surge; they are marathons that require persistence, patience, and the steady accumulation of small victories. This law reminds us that true progress is made through consistency and resilience, even when the steps seem small and the path long.

The Importance of Small Steps in Recovery

Trauma, whether it stems from war, abuse, or any other horrendous event, leaves deep imprints on the mind, body, and soul. These imprints manifest as crushing sensations, anxiety, depression, fear, nightmares, and an overwhelming sense of being out of control. The journey to recovery is not about erasing these memories—what has happened cannot be undone. Instead, it's about gradually reclaiming control over your life, step by step, by addressing the imprints of trauma and rebuilding your sense of self.

Recovery is about reestablishing ownership of your body and mind, which involves confronting the trauma and the emotions associated with it. This process cannot be rushed. If you dive too quickly into confronting the trauma without first building a foundation of safety and stability, you risk being retraumatized. Therefore, the first and most crucial step in recovery is learning to feel safe, calm, and focused.

Once a sense of safety is established, the journey continues with small, achievable goals: maintaining calm in the face of triggers, being present in the moment, and engaging fully with life again. These goals do not follow a strict sequence but often overlap, with some requiring more time and effort depending on individual circumstances. By focusing on small steps, you can build momentum and avoid feeling overwhelmed, reinforcing your progress one step at a time.

The Long March of Mao Zedong

A historical example that vividly illustrates the power of small steps is Mao Zedong's Long March. In 1934, during the Chinese Civil War, Mao and the Chinese Red Army were forced to retreat from their strongholds in southeastern China. Facing annihilation by the Nationalist forces, they embarked on what became known as the Long March—a journey of over 6,000 miles across treacherous terrain.

The Long March was not a single, bold stroke but a series of small, deliberate steps taken over a year. The Red Army faced constant danger from the elements, starvation, and attacks by the Nationalist forces. Yet, by breaking down the immense challenge into manageable segments, Mao led his forces through mountains, swamps, and deserts, all the while maintaining their morale and resilience.

The Long March became a symbol of perseverance and determination, demonstrating how seemingly insurmountable challenges can be overcome through the steady accumulation of small victories. The Red Army's survival and eventual success were not the result of one dramatic move but of thousands of small, strategic decisions and actions taken along the way.

Numerous studies in psychology and behavioral science support the idea that small, incremental steps are more effective for achieving long-term goals and recovery than attempting to make large, dramatic changes.

1. **Kaizen Principle**: The concept of "Kaizen," a Japanese term meaning "continuous improvement," is widely used in business and personal development. Research has shown that making small, incremental improvements is not only more sustainable but also leads to greater overall success. A study published in the *Harvard Business Review* highlighted how small, consistent changes lead to significant improvements in organizational performance over time. This principle can be directly applied to personal recovery and growth, where small, manageable changes accumulate to produce substantial long-term benefits.

2. **Behavioral Activation Therapy (BAT)**: In the field of mental health, particularly in the treatment of depression, Behavioral Activation Therapy (BAT) emphasizes the importance of small, achievable activities to break the cycle of avoidance and inactivity that often characterizes depression. Studies have shown that BAT, which encourages patients to engage in simple, pleasurable activities, can be as effective as cognitive-behavioral therapy (CBT) in treating depression. This approach demonstrates that small steps, like engaging in daily

activities, can significantly improve mental health and well-being.

3. **Micro-Goals and Motivation**: Research in motivation psychology suggests that setting small, achievable goals (micro-goals) enhances motivation and increases the likelihood of success. A study published in *Psychological Bulletin* found that breaking down goals into smaller, more manageable tasks reduces procrastination and helps individuals maintain focus and persistence. This supports the idea that conquering challenges through small steps builds momentum and reinforces progress.

4. **Neuroplasticity and Gradual Change**: Neuroscientific research on neuroplasticity—the brain's ability to reorganize itself by forming new neural connections—also supports the idea of small, consistent changes. Studies have shown that gradual, repetitive actions can lead to significant changes in the brain's structure and function, particularly in the areas related to learning and habit formation. This reinforces the notion that small steps can lead to profound changes in behavior and mental resilience over time.

Practical Steps To Achieving the 6th Law of Mental Power

To apply the sixth law of mental resilience in your own life, consider the following steps:

1. **Break Down the Challenge**: Start by breaking down the overwhelming task or challenge into smaller, manageable steps. Identify what needs to be done, and focus on one step at a time. This makes the process less intimidating and more achievable.

2. **Set Small, Achievable Goals**: Establish daily or weekly goals that are realistic and attainable. These should be steps that you can reasonably accomplish within a short

timeframe. Achieving these small goals will build your confidence and momentum.

3. **Celebrate Small Victories**: Acknowledge and celebrate each small victory along the way. Recognizing your progress, no matter how small, reinforces your efforts and motivates you to keep going.

4. **Be Patient and Persistent**: Understand that true progress is gradual. Be patient with yourself and persistent in your efforts. Even when progress seems slow, trust that each small step is bringing you closer to your goal.

5. **Stay Focused on the Present**: Focus on what you can do today rather than worrying about the entire journey ahead. Staying present helps prevent feelings of overwhelm and allows you to give your best effort to each step.

6. **Adjust as Needed**: Be flexible and willing to adjust your plan as needed. If a particular step is too difficult or not yielding the desired results, don't hesitate to reassess and find an alternative approach.

The sixth law of mental resilience, "Conquer in Small Steps," teaches us the value of gradual, consistent progress in overcoming life's challenges. By setting small, achievable goals and celebrating each step forward, we can build momentum and avoid feeling overwhelmed by the enormity of the tasks before us. Whether it's in recovering from trauma, achieving personal goals, or leading others through difficult times, this law reminds us that true progress is made one step at a time. Scientific research, historical examples like Mao Zedong's Long March, and psychological studies all support the effectiveness of this approach in building resilience and achieving lasting success.

Law 7

Control the Controllables

"It's not what happens to you, but how you react to it that matters." Epictetus

The seventh law of mental resilience, "Control the Controllables," is about focusing your energy on what you can influence—your actions, responses, and choices. In the aftermath of trauma, it's easy to feel as if your life is spiraling out of control, dictated by forces beyond your reach. But this law teaches us that true power lies in what we choose to control: our actions, our thoughts, and how we respond to the challenges life throws our way.

The Neuroscience Behind Trauma and Control

Imagine this: You're driving on a quiet road, the kind of journey that feels routine, almost automatic. You're chatting with a friend, the radio plays softly in the background, and everything feels normal—until, out of nowhere, a massive truck swerves into your lane. In an instant, your heart races, adrenaline floods your veins, and your body reacts faster than your mind can comprehend. You swerve to avoid the truck, narrowly escaping a crash, your heart pounding as the threat subsides.

This scenario is a perfect metaphor for how our brains handle trauma. The brain's amygdala, often called the "smoke detector," is responsible for alerting us to danger. It reacts swiftly and instinctively, just like you did when that truck appeared out of nowhere. But when trauma occurs, the amygdala goes into overdrive, becoming hypervigilant, and constantly on the lookout for threats. Meanwhile, the medial prefrontal cortex (MPFC), or the "watchtower," which helps us regulate our emotions and make rational decisions, becomes underactive. This imbalance can leave you feeling like you've lost control over your emotions and reactions.

Neuroimaging studies have shown that during episodes of intense fear, anger, or sadness—common in PTSD—subcortical regions of the brain associated with these emotions light up, while the frontal lobe, responsible for rational thought, dims down. It's as if the rational rider is trying to steer an unruly horse through a storm, desperately clinging on as the horse bucks and bolts in every direction.

But here's the crucial insight: While we may not be able to control the storm, we can learn to steady the horse and guide it through. This is where the concept of controlling the controllables comes into play. By focusing on what we can influence—our breathing, our thoughts, our responses—we can regain a sense of control, even in the midst of chaos.

Franklin D. Roosevelt and the Polio Epidemic

Let me take you back to 1921. Picture a vibrant, charismatic young man named Franklin D. Roosevelt, destined for greatness. At 39, he was already making waves in the political world, poised for a future that seemed limitless. But then, during a summer vacation, everything changed. Roosevelt was struck by a mysterious illness—polio—that left him paralyzed from the waist down.

Imagine the shock, the despair. Roosevelt, once full of energy and ambition, was now confined to a wheelchair, his dreams seemingly shattered. The doctors told him he would never walk again. He could have easily given in to despair, let the bitterness consume him, and resigned himself to a life defined by his limitations. But Roosevelt chose a different path. He chose to control what he could.

Roosevelt embarked on a grueling journey of rehabilitation, not just for himself, but for others who were similarly afflicted. He discovered Warm Springs, Georgia, a place with waters that seemed to offer relief to his paralyzed limbs. He bought the property and transformed it into a rehabilitation center, where he and others with polio could exercise, swim, and regain some measure of mobility. He didn't let his paralysis define him; instead, he focused on what he could do—strengthen his upper body, use braces to stand, and, perhaps most importantly, maintain his mind's sharpness and his spirit's indomitable will.

This determination, this focus on controlling the controllables, didn't just help Roosevelt physically; it transformed him mentally. It was during these years of struggle that he developed the resilience, empathy, and fortitude that would later guide him as he led the United States through the Great Depression and World War II. Roosevelt's story is not just one of overcoming adversity; it's a testament to the power of focusing on what you can control, even when the world seems to be falling apart.

Research Supporting the Importance of Focusing on Controllables

1. **Locus of Control**: Psychologist Julian Rotter's theory of "locus of control" explores how individuals perceive their ability to influence outcomes. Those with an internal locus of control believe they have the power to shape their destiny through their actions. Studies have shown that these individuals are more resilient, less likely to suffer

from anxiety or depression, and better equipped to handle stress. They know that while they cannot control everything, they can control their response to what happens.

2. **Mindfulness and Emotional Regulation**: Mindfulness practices have gained widespread recognition for their ability to help individuals control their responses to stress and trauma. A study published in *JAMA Internal Medicine* found that veterans with PTSD who practiced mindfulness experienced significant reductions in symptoms. Mindfulness helps bring the "watchtower" back online, allowing individuals to observe their thoughts and feelings without being overwhelmed by them.

3. **Cognitive Behavioral Therapy (CBT)**: CBT is another powerful tool that aligns with this law. It teaches individuals to recognize and challenge unhelpful thoughts and behaviors, focusing on what they can change. A comprehensive review published in *The Lancet Psychiatry* confirmed that CBT is highly effective in treating anxiety, depression, and PTSD. By controlling their thoughts and responses, individuals can reshape their experience of reality.

How to Achieve the Seventh Law: Practical Steps

To apply the seventh law of mental resilience in your own life, consider the following strategies:

1. **Identify What You Can Control**: In any situation, start by identifying the aspects you can influence. Focus your energy on these areas, rather than on what is beyond your control. This might include your actions, your attitude, and your reactions to external events.

2. **Practice Mindfulness**: Incorporate mindfulness into your daily routine. Whether through meditation, deep

breathing exercises, or simply paying attention to your thoughts, mindfulness helps you stay grounded and focused on what you can control.

3. **Strengthen Emotional Regulation**: Use techniques like controlled breathing, yoga, or physical exercise to help regulate your emotions. These practices help calm the "smoke detector" and strengthen the "watchtower," allowing you to respond rather than react.

4. **Set Realistic Goals**: Establish small, achievable goals that focus on areas where you have control. This approach helps build momentum and gives you a sense of accomplishment, reinforcing your sense of agency.

5. **Seek Support When Needed**: If you find it difficult to manage your emotions or control your responses, don't hesitate to seek support. Therapies like CBT can provide you with strategies to regain control over your thoughts and behaviors.

The seventh law of mental resilience, "Control the Controllables," teaches us that while we cannot control everything in life, we can control how we respond to what happens. By focusing on what we can influence—our actions, thoughts, and emotions—we regain a sense of power and agency, even in the face of trauma and adversity. Franklin D. Roosevelt's story, along with scientific research, underscores the effectiveness of this approach. By applying this law, you can navigate life's challenges with greater confidence and resilience, transforming obstacles into opportunities for growth.

Law 8

Find Your Escape

"Imagination is everything. It is the preview of life's coming attractions." Albert Einstein

The eighth law of mental resilience, "Find Your Escape," underscores the importance of having healthy outlets to cope with stress and maintain mental well-being. Life's challenges, especially those stemming from trauma, can overwhelm even the strongest individuals, making it crucial to have effective coping mechanisms that allow you to process emotions and reduce stress. Healthy escapes such as exercise, journaling, or creative outlets offer productive ways to navigate the intensity of your feelings and regain your sense of balance.

The Science Behind Healthy Escapes

From a young age, children instinctively develop coping mechanisms based on their interactions with caregivers. These early coping styles can have long-lasting effects on how individuals manage stress and emotions throughout their lives. Research conducted by Mary Ainsworth and Mary Main on attachment styles provides critical insights into how these coping mechanisms form and evolve.

Ainsworth's "Strange Situation" study demonstrated that securely attached infants, who experience consistent and responsive care, are more likely to develop healthy ways of dealing with stress. On the other hand, children with insecure attachments often adopt maladaptive coping strategies. For example, those with avoidant attachment may seem indifferent to stress but actually suffer from chronic hyperarousal, while those with anxious attachment may become excessively clingy or emotionally volatile. These early coping styles often persist into adulthood, affecting how people respond to stress and trauma.

However, even those who develop maladaptive coping strategies in childhood can learn healthier ways to manage their emotions. Neuroscience has shown that engaging in healthy coping mechanisms can help regulate the brain's response to stress. Activities like exercise, creative expression, and mindfulness practice engage the brain's prefrontal cortex, helping to calm the amygdala—the brain's "smoke detector"—and reducing the intensity of emotional responses. By finding a healthy escape, individuals can better manage their stress and avoid being overwhelmed by negative emotions.

Winston Churchill and the "Black Dog"

A compelling historical example of the power of finding a healthy escape is found in the life of Winston Churchill, the British Prime Minister during World War II. Churchill was known not only for his leadership during one of the darkest times in modern history but also for his lifelong struggle with depression, which he referred to as his "black dog."

Churchill's battle with depression was intense and persistent. He often faced dark moods that left him feeling isolated and despairing. Despite these challenges, Churchill found solace and strength in several healthy escapes that helped him manage his mental health and maintain his resilience in the face of overwhelming adversity.

One of Churchill's most significant escapes was painting. He discovered this hobby later in life, during a particularly difficult period following a political setback. For Churchill, painting provided a much-needed break from the pressures of public life. The act of creating something beautiful allowed him to momentarily step away from his worries and immerse himself in a world of color and form. It was more than just a distraction; it was a way to process his emotions and regain his mental equilibrium.

Churchill also found refuge in writing. Throughout his life, he wrote prolifically, not only as a means of communication but also as a therapeutic outlet. His writings, including his memoirs and speeches, helped him articulate his thoughts, process his emotions, and leave a legacy that would inspire future generations.

These healthy escapes were crucial in helping Churchill manage his "black dog" and remain resilient during some of the most challenging moments in history. His ability to find solace in creative outlets played a significant role in his mental health, allowing him to lead with strength and clarity when the world needed him most.

Research Supporting Healthy Escapes

1. **Exercise and Mental Health**: Numerous studies have demonstrated the positive effects of physical activity on mental health. Exercise has been shown to reduce symptoms of depression and anxiety by boosting endorphins and improving brain function. A study published in the *American Journal of Psychiatry* found that regular physical activity significantly reduced the risk of developing depression, highlighting the importance of exercise as a healthy escape.

2. **Journaling and Emotional Processing**: Writing about emotions, often referred to as expressive writing or journaling, has been shown to have therapeutic effects. A study published in *Psychosomatic Medicine* found that individuals who engaged in expressive writing experienced lower levels of stress and improved immune function. Journaling provides a safe space to explore and process complex emotions, making it an effective coping mechanism for dealing with stress and trauma.

3. **Creative Expression and Brain Function**: Engaging in creative activities such as painting, music, or dance can have profound effects on mental health. Research published in *The Arts in Psychotherapy* has shown that creative expression helps reduce stress, enhance mood, and improve cognitive function. Creative outlets activate areas of the brain associated with pleasure and reward, providing a healthy escape that can counterbalance the effects of stress and negative emotions.

How to Achieve the Eighth Law: Practical Steps

To apply the eighth law of mental resilience, "Find Your Escape," in your own life, consider the following strategies:

1. **Identify Your Healthy Escapes**: Reflect on activities that bring you joy, relaxation, or a sense of accomplishment. Whether it's exercise, journaling, painting, or playing music, find an activity that allows you to step away from your stress and engage in something that nourishes your soul.

2. **Incorporate These Activities into Your Routine**: Make time for your healthy escapes regularly. This could mean setting aside time each day for a short walk, journaling before bed, or dedicating a weekend afternoon to your creative hobby. Consistency is key to reaping the benefits of these activities.

3. **Use Escapes as a Tool for Emotional Regulation**: Recognize when you're feeling overwhelmed or stressed and turn to your healthy escapes as a way to process those emotions. These activities can serve as a safe space where you can express your feelings and regain your emotional balance.

4. **Experiment with New Outlets**: If you're not sure what your healthy escape might be, don't be afraid to experiment. Try different activities to see what resonates with you. The goal is to find something that feels both enjoyable and therapeutic.

5. **Balance Escapism with Reality**: While healthy escapes are important, it's also essential to balance them with facing and addressing the issues at hand. Use your escapes as a way to recharge and gain perspective, but also ensure that you're taking steps to deal with the underlying causes of your stress or emotions.

The eighth law of mental resilience, "Find Your Escape," emphasizes the importance of having healthy outlets to manage stress and process emotions. Through examples like Winston Churchill's use of painting and writing to combat his "black dog," and supported by extensive research on the benefits of exercise, journaling, and creative expression, this law underscores the power of productive escapes in maintaining mental health. By identifying and incorporating healthy escapes into your routine, you can build resilience, reduce stress, and find a sanctuary for your mind amidst the challenges of life.

Law 9

Stay Present

"If you are depressed, you are living in the past. If you are anxious, you are living in the future. If you are at peace, you are living in the present." Lao Tzu

The ninth law of mental resilience, "Stay Present," reminds us that the past is a shadow, the future a mirage, and that only the present moment is real. For those who have experienced trauma, this simple truth can be incredibly difficult to grasp. Trauma often roots us in the past, replaying painful memories over and over again, or catapults us into the future, filling us with anxiety about what might happen next. However, learning to stay grounded in the present through mindfulness practices can help loosen the grip of traumatic memories and future worries, allowing us to find peace in the here and now.

Understanding Trauma and the Power of the Present

Since the early 1990s, advancements in brain imaging have provided profound insights into the impact of trauma on the brain and body. We now understand that trauma isn't just an event that happened in the past; it's an experience that leaves a deep imprint on the mind, brain, and body, affecting how we perceive and interact with the world long after the event itself has passed.

Trauma fundamentally reorganizes the brain's way of managing perceptions. It alters not only our thoughts but our very capacity to think, often leaving us stuck in a state of hypervigilance— constantly on alert for danger that may never come. This heightened state of arousal is not merely psychological; it's deeply physical. The body remains on edge, ready to react to perceived threats, even when there are none. The challenge for those who have been traumatized is to teach their bodies and minds that the danger is over and that they are safe in the present moment.

Simply recounting traumatic experiences, while important, is not enough to heal. Words alone cannot override the automatic, deeply ingrained responses of a body that has been conditioned by trauma to remain in a state of constant readiness. Real healing requires a shift in how the body and mind perceive the present, learning to recognize that the present moment is safe and that the past no longer holds power over them.

Emily was a 32-year-old graphic designer living in a bustling city. On the surface, she had it all: a successful career, a close-knit group of friends, and a cozy apartment in a neighborhood she loved. But beneath this exterior, Emily was struggling with something that had haunted her for years.

Seven years earlier, Emily had been involved in a serious car accident. She was driving home one evening when another driver, distracted by their phone, ran a red light and crashed into her car. Emily was left with multiple injuries, but the physical scars weren't the worst part. The trauma of the accident lingered long after her body had healed. She couldn't stop reliving the moment of impact, the screeching tires, the sound of shattering glass, and the jolt of pain. The memory played in her mind like a loop, pulling her back to that terrifying night every time she got behind the wheel or even heard a loud noise.

As time passed, Emily became increasingly anxious about driving, and soon, she was avoiding it altogether. She relied on public transportation or her friends to get around. The thought of being in another accident was too much to bear, and even though she knew it was irrational, she couldn't shake the feeling that something terrible was going to happen again. Her mind was stuck in the past, replaying the trauma, while also projecting those fears into the future, imagining all the ways things could go wrong.

The stress began to take its toll. Emily started experiencing panic attacks, which made her feel even more out of control. Her work began to suffer, and she withdrew from social activities, preferring to stay in the safety of her apartment. She felt trapped, unable to escape the past or the anxiety about what might come next.

One day, after a particularly intense panic attack, Emily decided she couldn't go on like this. She reached out to a therapist who specialized in trauma and mindfulness-based practices. Her therapist introduced her to mindfulness techniques designed to help her stay present, rather than being dragged into the past or worrying about the future.

At first, mindfulness seemed almost too simple to be effective. Her therapist guided her through exercises like focusing on her breath, observing her thoughts without judgment, and paying attention to the sensations in her body. Emily practiced these techniques daily, even when she didn't feel like it. Slowly, she began to notice a shift.

One afternoon, while sitting in her apartment, Emily felt the familiar wave of anxiety start to rise. Her heart raced, and her mind began to spiral into "what ifs"—what if she had another panic attack? What if she lost control? But this time, instead of getting swept away by the fear, she focused on her breath, feeling the air move in and out of her lungs. She brought her attention to the present moment, grounding herself in the sensations around her— the softness of the couch, the warmth of the sunlight streaming through the window, the steady rhythm of her breath.

As she did this, the anxiety didn't disappear completely, but it began to lose its grip. For the first time in years, Emily realized that she could stay present, that the past was not happening now, and that the future was not something she had to fear at this moment. She was safe, right here, right now.

With continued practice, Emily's panic attacks became less frequent and less intense. She still had moments of fear, but she learned to bring herself back to the present, using the mindfulness techniques she had practiced. She even began driving again, starting with short trips and gradually building up her confidence. By staying present, she was able to reclaim her life from the trauma that had held her captive for so long.

Research Supporting Mindfulness and Staying Present

1. **Mindfulness and Trauma Recovery**: Research shows that mindfulness practices, which focus on staying present and observing thoughts and sensations without judgment, are highly effective in trauma recovery. A study in *The Journal of Traumatic Stress* found that mindfulness-based stress reduction (MBSR) significantly reduced symptoms of PTSD, helping individuals shift their focus from the past or future to the present moment.

2. **Neuroscience of Mindfulness**: Neuroimaging studies demonstrate that mindfulness can change brain structure and function. A study published in *Psychiatry Research: Neuroimaging* found that mindfulness meditation increased gray matter density in the hippocampus, a

region involved in memory and emotional regulation, and reduced activity in the amygdala, the brain's fear center. These changes suggest that mindfulness helps the brain become less reactive to stress and more anchored in the present.

3. **Psychological Well-being and the Present Moment**: A study in *Psychological Science* found that people who spend more time focusing on the present moment tend to be happier and less anxious. When the mind wanders to the past or future, people generally feel less happy. Staying present helps individuals engage fully with their current experiences, leading to greater overall well-being.

How to Achieve the Ninth Law: Practical Steps

To apply the ninth law of mental resilience, "Stay Present," in your own life, consider the following strategies:

1. **Practice Mindfulness Daily**: Incorporate mindfulness practices into your daily routine. Focus on your breath, observe your thoughts, or pay attention to the sensations in your body. The key is to stay present with whatever is happening in the moment, without judgment or attachment.

2. **Ground Yourself in the Present**: When you find yourself ruminating on the past or worrying about the future, bring your attention back to the present moment. Use grounding techniques, such as focusing on the physical sensations of your body, describing your surroundings in detail, or engaging in a simple task like washing dishes or walking.

3. **Engage in Present-Focused Activities**: Engage in activities that naturally bring you into the present moment, such as yoga, meditation, or creative pursuits like painting or playing an instrument. These activities require your full

attention and can help you stay grounded in the here and now.

4. **Limit Time Spent on Unproductive Thoughts**: Set boundaries on how much time you spend thinking about the past or future. While reflection and planning are important, excessive rumination or anxiety can be counterproductive. Practice redirecting your thoughts back to the present when you notice they've wandered.

5. **Seek Professional Support if Needed**: If staying present is particularly challenging due to trauma or chronic anxiety, consider seeking support from a therapist who specializes in mindfulness-based therapies or trauma-informed care. Professional guidance can provide you with additional tools and techniques to help you stay grounded.

The ninth law of mental resilience, "Stay Present," emphasizes the importance of anchoring yourself in the present moment to break free from the grip of past traumas and future anxieties. Emily's story illustrates how mindfulness practices can help regain control and find peace in the present, even after experiencing profound trauma. Supported by extensive research on mindfulness and its impact on the brain, this law reminds us that true peace and resilience are found in fully embracing the present. By practicing mindfulness and staying grounded in the now, you can cultivate the mental strength needed to navigate life's ups and downs with grace and stability.

Law 10

Create Rituals

"We are what we repeatedly do. Excellence, then, is not an act, but a habit." Aristotle

The tenth law of mental resilience, "Create Rituals," underscores the importance of routines and rituals in providing stability, especially in the chaotic aftermath of trauma. Routines serve as anchors, offering a sense of normalcy and grounding in times when everything else seems uncertain. Whether it's a morning coffee ritual, daily exercise, or meditation, establishing these practices can help you regain control and create a structured environment that fosters mental well-being.

The Power of Rituals: From Ancient Times to Today

Since the dawn of civilization, humans have relied on rituals to cope with their most powerful and terrifying emotions. Ancient Greek theater, one of the earliest forms of communal ritual, evolved from religious rites that involved dancing, singing, and reenacting mythical stories. By the fifth century BCE, theater had become a central part of civic life in Greece, particularly in Athens, where performances were often attended by veterans of war.

These performances, such as the tragedies written by Aeschylus and Sophocles, served as a form of ritual reintegration for combat veterans. The themes explored in these plays—betrayal, loss, revenge, and forgiveness—mirrored the inner turmoil of those who had witnessed and participated in the horrors of war. The communal experience of watching these plays, where the audience could see each other's emotions and reactions, helped veterans process their trauma collectively. This ancient form of ritualized storytelling provided a safe space for individuals to confront their deepest fears and emotions, allowing them to reintegrate into society with a renewed sense of purpose and understanding.

In modern times, rituals continue to play a crucial role in helping individuals navigate trauma and stress. Neuroscientific research has shown that routines and rituals can positively affect the brain, particularly in areas related to stress management and emotional regulation. By engaging in regular rituals, individuals can create a predictable and safe environment, which is essential for maintaining mental resilience in the face of adversity.

The Power of Ritual in Nelson Mandela's Life

Referring back to the story of Nelson Mandela from the Fourth Law, one of the most powerful examples of the impact of ritual can be found in his 27 years of imprisonment on Robben Island. Mandela, who would go on to become South Africa's first Black president, was incarcerated for his unwavering resistance to apartheid. During his imprisonment, he endured brutal conditions—physical labor, isolation, and severely restricted contact with the outside world. Despite these hardships, Mandela's commitment to daily rituals played a crucial role in sustaining his resilience and preserving his sense of purpose throughout those long years.

Despite these challenges, Mandela maintained his mental resilience by creating and adhering to daily rituals. Every morning, he would wake up early to exercise, even in the cramped and inhospitable conditions of his cell. This ritual was not just about physical fitness; it was a way for Mandela to assert control over his environment and maintain his dignity in the face of dehumanizing circumstances.

In addition to physical exercise, Mandela established rituals around his intellectual and spiritual development. He requested books and engaged in regular reading and writing, which allowed him to continue his education and stay connected to the broader world. These rituals provided structure to his day, offering a sense of normalcy and purpose that helped him endure the long years of imprisonment.

Mandela's commitment to his rituals also had a communal impact. He encouraged his fellow prisoners to adopt similar practices, fostering a sense of solidarity and mutual support among them. These shared rituals helped the prisoners maintain their mental and emotional well-being, creating a collective resilience that sustained them throughout their ordeal.

Mandela's ability to create and adhere to rituals during one of the most challenging periods of his life illustrates the profound impact that routines can have on mental resilience. His story serves as a powerful reminder that even in the most adverse conditions, rituals can provide a sense of control, stability, and hope.

Research Supporting the Importance of Rituals

1. **The Neuroscience of Rituals**: Research in neuroscience has shown that rituals can have a calming effect on the brain. A study published in *Social Cognitive and Affective Neuroscience* found that engaging in rituals can reduce anxiety and stress by activating the brain's reward system. Rituals help create a sense of predictability and control,

which is crucial for managing stress and maintaining mental resilience.

2. **Rituals and Psychological Stability**: A study published in the *Journal of Clinical Psychology* found that individuals who engage in daily rituals, such as morning routines or bedtime rituals, report higher levels of psychological stability and well-being. These rituals provide a sense of structure and routine, which can be especially beneficial in times of chaos or uncertainty.

3. **Collective Rituals and Social Bonding**: Research published in *Behavioral and Brain Sciences* highlights the role of collective rituals in fostering social cohesion and resilience. Rituals that involve communal participation, such as religious ceremonies, group exercises, or even shared meals, help strengthen social bonds and create a sense of belonging. This collective bonding can be particularly important in helping individuals cope with trauma and stress.

How to Achieve the Tenth Law: Practical Steps

To apply the tenth law of mental resilience, "Create Rituals," in your own life, consider the following strategies:

1. **Establish Daily Rituals**: Identify daily activities that bring you a sense of calm and stability. This could be something as simple as making your morning coffee, going for a walk, or practicing meditation. Incorporate these activities into your daily routine to create a sense of normalcy and structure.

2. **Create Meaningful Rituals**: Beyond daily routines, consider creating rituals that hold personal significance. For example, you might develop a ritual around journaling at the end of each day, lighting a candle before meditation, or practicing gratitude during meals. These rituals can help

you connect with your values and provide a deeper sense of purpose.

3. **Engage in Collective Rituals**: Whenever possible, participate in collective rituals that foster social connection. This could include attending religious services, joining a community group, or simply sharing a meal with loved ones. Collective rituals can strengthen your sense of belonging and provide additional support during challenging times.

4. **Adapt Rituals to Changing Circumstances**: Life is unpredictable, and circumstances may change. Be flexible with your rituals, allowing them to evolve as needed. The key is to maintain a sense of routine and structure, even if the specific activities change.

5. **Use Rituals as Anchors During Stress**: When you're feeling overwhelmed or stressed, turn to your rituals as a way to ground yourself. These routines can provide a sense of stability and control, helping you navigate difficult emotions and situations with greater resilience.

The tenth law of mental resilience, "Create Rituals," emphasizes the importance of routines in providing stability and grounding, especially in the chaotic aftermath of trauma. From the ancient Greek theater to Nelson Mandela's daily rituals in prison, history is rich with examples of how rituals can help individuals and communities navigate adversity. Supported by research in neuroscience and psychology, this law reminds us that rituals are powerful tools for maintaining mental resilience. By establishing and adhering to meaningful rituals, you can create a sense of normalcy, control, and purpose that will sustain you through life's challenges.

Law 11

Prioritize Rest

"Sleep is that golden chain that ties health and our bodies together." Thomas Dekker

Rest is not a luxury; it's a critical component of mental resilience and healing, especially in the aftermath of trauma. The eleventh law of mental resilience, "Prioritize Rest," emphasizes the importance of sleep as a foundation for recovery. Trauma disrupts the body's ability to rest and recover, leading to a host of physical and psychological challenges. By prioritizing sleep, you allow your body and mind the opportunity to heal, regenerate, and build the resilience needed to face life's challenges.

The Science Behind Rest and Recovery

The brain's primary function is to ensure our survival, constantly monitoring and managing our body's needs. Sleep is one of the most fundamental of these needs. It is during sleep that the brain processes and integrates experiences repairs cellular damage, and regulates emotions. However, trauma can severely disrupt sleep patterns, leading to insomnia, nightmares, and chronic fatigue. Without adequate rest, the brain struggles to perform these essential functions, leaving the body and mind in a state of perpetual stress and imbalance.

The brain is composed of several layers, each with a specific role in maintaining our well-being. The most primitive part, known as the reptilian brain, controls basic survival functions such as breathing, eating, and sleeping. When sleep is disrupted, these basic functions are thrown into disarray, affecting everything from mood to immune function.

The limbic system, or mammalian brain, is responsible for processing emotions and managing our responses to stress. Trauma can overstimulate the limbic system, making it difficult to regulate emotions and leading to problems like anxiety and depression. Sleep is essential for calming the limbic system and restoring emotional balance.

Finally, the neocortex, our rational brain, is responsible for higher-order functions like decision-making, problem-solving, and planning. Sleep deprivation impairs these cognitive functions, making it harder to process trauma and make sound decisions. Prioritizing rest ensures that the neocortex can function effectively, supporting mental clarity and resilience.

The Difference in Healing: Rest vs. No Rest

Let's visualize the impact of prioritizing rest on healing, using a chart that compares the recovery outcomes between those who prioritize rest and those who do not.

Aspect of Healing	Prioritize Rest	Neglect Rest
Emotional Regulation	Improved emotional stability and reduced anxiety.	Increased emotional volatility and heightened anxiety.
Cognitive Function	Enhanced problem-solving, memory consolidation, and decision-making.	Impaired cognitive abilities, poor memory, and decision-making

		difficulties.
Physical Health	Stronger immune function, reduced inflammation, and faster physical recovery.	Weakened immune system, increased inflammation, and slower recovery.
Trauma Recovery	Better processing and integration of traumatic memories, leading to reduced PTSD symptoms.	Persistent PTSD symptoms, difficulty processing trauma, and prolonged recovery.
Overall Well-Being	Increased resilience, mental clarity, and a greater sense of control.	Decreased resilience, mental fog, and a sense of overwhelm.

This chart illustrates the stark difference in healing outcomes between individuals who prioritize rest and those who do not. Those who prioritize sleep experience better emotional regulation, cognitive function, physical health, and trauma recovery, all of which contribute to overall well-being and mental resilience.

Winston Churchill and the Power of Napping

Winston Churchill, the iconic British Prime Minister during World War II, is a prime example of how prioritizing rest can bolster mental resilience in even the most stressful situations. Despite the immense pressures of leading a nation at war, Churchill made it a point to take a nap every afternoon. He believed that this ritual was crucial for maintaining his mental clarity and stamina, allowing him to make sound decisions during the long and grueling days of the war.

Churchill's commitment to rest didn't just benefit him personally; it also influenced those around him. By modeling the importance of rest, he encouraged his staff and military leaders to do the same, fostering a culture of resilience and sustained effort. Churchill's ability to balance intense work with regular rest was a key factor in his effective leadership and the eventual success of his nation.

How to Prioritize Rest: Practical Steps

To apply the eleventh law of mental resilience in your life, consider the following steps:

1. **Establish a Consistent Sleep Routine**: Set a regular sleep schedule by going to bed and waking up at the same time every day. Consistency helps regulate your body's internal clock and improves sleep quality.

2. **Create a Sleep-Conducive Environment**: Optimize your sleep environment by keeping your bedroom cool, dark, and quiet. Invest in a comfortable mattress and pillows to ensure physical comfort during sleep.

3. **Practice Pre-Sleep Relaxation**: Engage in relaxing activities before bed, such as reading, taking a warm bath, or practicing deep breathing exercises. These activities help calm your mind and prepare your body for restful sleep.

4. **Limit Stimulants Before Bedtime**: Avoid caffeine, nicotine, and heavy meals in the hours leading up to bedtime, as these can interfere with your ability to fall asleep.

5. **Incorporate Short Naps When Needed**: If you're feeling fatigued during the day, consider taking a short nap (20-30 minutes) to recharge. However, avoid napping too close to bedtime to prevent disruptions to your nighttime sleep.

6. **Seek Professional Help for Persistent Sleep Issues**: If trauma or stress is severely affecting your sleep, consider seeking help from a therapist or sleep specialist. Cognitive

Behavioral Therapy for Insomnia (CBT-I) is an effective treatment that can help improve sleep quality and manage trauma-related sleep disturbances.

The eleventh law of mental resilience, "Prioritize Rest," highlights the indispensable role of sleep in the healing process. Trauma can disrupt the body's natural ability to rest and recover, but by prioritizing sleep, you allow your brain and body to heal, regenerate, and restore balance. The contrast between those who prioritize rest and those who neglect it is clear: rest leads to improved emotional regulation, cognitive function, physical health, and overall resilience. By adopting a consistent sleep routine, creating a restful environment, and practicing relaxation techniques, you can ensure that your mind and body are equipped to handle life's challenges with strength and clarity.

Law 12

Feed the Mind, Feed the Body

"Let food be thy medicine and medicine be thy food." Hippocrates

"What nourishes you sustains you—inside and out." This twelfth law of mental resilience highlights the critical connection between nutrition and mental health. Just as our bodies require a balanced diet to function optimally, so too does our mind. The food we consume directly impacts our mood, energy levels, and emotional stability, all of which are vital components of the healing process, particularly after experiencing trauma. By nourishing both the mind and body, we create a strong foundation for recovery and resilience.

The Science Behind Nutrition and Mental Health

Our understanding of the profound impact of nutrition on mental health has deepened significantly in recent years. The emerging field of nutritional psychiatry explores how diet influences mental well-being, revealing that the foods we eat play a crucial role in brain function and emotional regulation.

The brain is an incredibly energy-hungry organ, consuming about 20% of the body's total energy. To maintain optimal function, it requires a steady supply of nutrients, including vitamins, minerals, amino acids, and fatty acids. These nutrients are essential for producing neurotransmitters—the chemicals that transmit signals between nerve cells. For example, serotonin, often referred to as the "feel-good" neurotransmitter, is synthesized from the amino acid tryptophan, which is found in foods like turkey, nuts, and seeds. A deficiency in these essential nutrients can lead to imbalances in neurotransmitter levels, contributing to mood disorders such as depression and anxiety.

Moreover, the gut-brain connection underscores the importance of nutrition in mental health. The gut, often called the "second brain," contains a vast network of neurons and produces many of the same neurotransmitters as the brain, including serotonin. A healthy gut microbiome—supported by a diet rich in fiber, fruits, vegetables, and fermented foods—promotes better mental health by reducing inflammation and improving neurotransmitter production.

The Role of Nutrition in World War II Recovery

A historical example that vividly illustrates the power of nutrition in mental and physical recovery is the post-World War II recovery effort. After the devastation of the war, many populations, particularly in Europe, were left malnourished and weakened, both physically and mentally. The Marshall Plan, initiated by the United States, was not only an economic recovery program but also a comprehensive effort to restore health through improved nutrition.

As part of the Marshall Plan, there was a significant focus on addressing malnutrition among European populations. Food supplies were distributed, and nutritional programs were established to help rebuild the health of millions of people. Studies conducted during this period showed that improved nutrition led to significant improvements in mental health outcomes, particularly among children who had been severely affected by the war.

One striking example is the Dutch Famine of 1944-1945, also known as the "Hunger Winter," where the population of the Netherlands experienced extreme food shortages. Children who were born during or immediately after this famine were found to have higher rates of mental health issues later in life, including depression and schizophrenia. However, those who received adequate nutrition during the early post-war years showed better mental health outcomes, underscoring the critical role of nutrition in recovery from trauma.

The Impact of Diet on Mental Health: Research and Statistics

Research in nutritional psychiatry provides compelling evidence that diet plays a crucial role in mental health:

1. **The Mediterranean Diet**: A study published in *BMC Medicine* found that individuals who followed a Mediterranean diet—rich in fruits, vegetables, whole grains, nuts, and olive oil—had a 30% lower risk of developing depression compared to those who followed a Western diet high in processed foods and refined sugars. The anti-inflammatory properties of the Mediterranean diet, along with its high levels of essential nutrients, contribute to its protective effects on mental health.

2. **Omega-3 Fatty Acids**: Omega-3 fatty acids, found in fish like salmon and sardines, as well as in flaxseeds and walnuts, have been shown to reduce symptoms of depression and anxiety. A meta-analysis published in *Translational Psychiatry* revealed that supplementation with omega-3 fatty acids significantly improved depressive symptoms in individuals with major depressive disorder.

3. **Gut Health and Mental Health**: A study published in *Molecular Psychiatry* demonstrated the link between gut health and mental health. Researchers found that individuals with a healthy gut microbiome were less likely to experience anxiety and depression. The study highlighted the importance of a diet rich in prebiotics and probiotics, such as those found in fiber-rich foods and fermented products, in maintaining mental well-being.

4. **Sugar and Mood**: High consumption of refined sugars has been linked to increased risks of depression and mood disorders. A study published in *Scientific Reports* found that individuals who consumed diets high in added sugars were more likely to develop depression over time. The study suggests that reducing sugar intake and replacing it with nutrient-dense foods can lead to better mental health outcomes.

How to Achieve the Twelfth Law: Practical Steps

To apply the twelfth law of mental resilience, "Feed the Mind, Feed the Body," in your own life, consider the following strategies:

1. **Adopt a Balanced Diet**: Focus on a diet rich in whole foods, including plenty of fruits, vegetables, whole grains, lean proteins, and healthy fats. The Mediterranean diet is an excellent model to follow, as it is associated with numerous mental health benefits.

2. **Incorporate Omega-3 Fatty Acids**: Include sources of omega-3 fatty acids in your diet, such as fatty fish (e.g., salmon, mackerel), flaxseeds, chia seeds, and walnuts. These nutrients support brain health and help regulate mood.

3. **Support Gut Health**: Eat a diet that supports a healthy gut microbiome by incorporating fiber-rich foods, such as

fruits, vegetables, and whole grains, as well as fermented foods like yogurt, kefir, sauerkraut, and kimchi.

4. **Limit Processed Foods and Sugars**: Reduce your intake of processed foods and added sugars, which can contribute to inflammation and negatively impact mental health. Opt for natural sweeteners like honey or maple syrup in moderation.

5. **Stay Hydrated**: Hydration is essential for overall health, including mental clarity and mood regulation. Aim to drink plenty of water throughout the day to stay hydrated and support your body's functions.

6. **Consider Nutritional Supplements**: If you have specific dietary restrictions or are unable to obtain certain nutrients through food alone, consider taking supplements such as omega-3s, vitamin D, or B vitamins, after consulting with a healthcare provider.

The twelfth law of mental resilience, "Feed the Mind, Feed the Body," emphasizes the critical role of nutrition in maintaining mental health and fostering recovery from trauma. Historical examples like the post-World War II recovery efforts and contemporary research in nutritional psychiatry demonstrate that what we eat profoundly impacts our mood, energy levels, and emotional stability. By adopting a balanced diet rich in whole foods, supporting gut health, and limiting processed foods, you can nourish both your mind and body, creating a strong foundation for mental resilience and overall well-being.

Law 13

Move to Heal

"Take care of your body. It's the only place you have to live." Jim Rohn

"Physical movement is a balm for a weary mind." This law captures the profound impact that physical activity can have on healing, especially for those who have experienced trauma. When trauma strikes, it often traps stress and tension within the body, manifesting as chronic anxiety, hypervigilance, or a sense of being emotionally numb. Physical movement offers a powerful way to release this trapped energy, reconnect the mind and body, and promote overall well-being.

A Personal Journey: Rediscovering Movement After Trauma

I still remember the day I walked into the trauma center for the first time. The air was heavy with silence, punctuated by the occasional murmur of conversations and the distant hum of a coffee machine. I had been through months of therapy, trying to make sense of the anxiety that gripped me every morning, the nightmares that left me drenched in sweat, and the overwhelming sense of being stuck in my own body. But despite the countless hours spent talking through my experiences, something still felt off—like I was missing a key piece of the puzzle.

The waiting room was full of people like me, each carrying their own invisible burdens. But among them was Steve, a staff member who seemed to have an energy that cut through the somber atmosphere. He wasn't a therapist in the traditional sense—no notepad, no probing questions. Instead, he carried a brightly colored beach ball, of all things. At first, I thought it was a bit childish, almost out of place in such a serious setting. But Steve didn't seem to care about how it looked.

He noticed me sitting in the corner, arms crossed tightly, trying to hold myself together. Without a word, he tossed the ball toward me. It landed by my feet, and I stared at it, unsure of what to do. Steve just smiled, his eyes inviting me to play along. I hesitated—part of me wanted to ignore him, to stay wrapped up in the familiar cocoon of my anxiety. But something about his approach was disarming. I nudged the ball back with my foot, a small, tentative push.

To my surprise, it felt good. It wasn't much, just a gentle kick, but it was enough to shift something inside me. Steve caught the ball and sent it back, this time a little harder. We began a slow, back-and-forth game, no words exchanged, just the rhythm of the ball bouncing between us. And with each pass, I felt a little more of the tension ease out of my body as if the movement was shaking loose the fear that had taken root inside me.

That was the first time I realized that healing didn't have to come through words alone. There was something about the physical act of moving—of engaging my body—that spoke to a part of me that therapy hadn't yet reached.

The Healing Power of Physical Movement

Steve's approach wasn't just about playing with a ball. It was about reawakening a part of myself that had been dormant since the trauma. Trauma often leaves us stuck in a state of hyperarousal or shutdown, where our bodies remain on high alert or completely numb to the world around us. Movement helps to break through those barriers, offering a way to release the stress and tension that's been stored deep within our muscles and tissues.

Over the next few weeks, I found myself drawn to the more physical aspects of the trauma center's program. There was a yoga class, specifically designed for trauma survivors, that became a lifeline for me. The first time I walked into the studio, I was skeptical. I had tried yoga before, but it had always felt like a performance—something I was doing to look good or to fit in. But this was different.

The instructor, a gentle woman with a calming presence, guided us through the movements with a focus on how they felt, rather than how they looked. She encouraged us to listen to our bodies, to notice the sensations that arose, and to move in ways that felt safe and comfortable. It wasn't about pushing ourselves or achieving perfect poses—it was about reconnecting with our bodies in a way that felt healing.

There was one pose, in particular, that became my favorite—a child's pose. It's a simple, restorative pose, where you kneel on the floor and fold forward, resting your forehead on the mat. The first time I tried it, I felt a wave of emotion wash over me. I hadn't realized how disconnected I had been from my own body until that moment. As I breathed deeply, feeling the stretch in my back and the gentle pressure of the mat against my forehead, I felt something release inside me. It was as if I was finally permitting myself to let go, to stop holding everything so tightly.

The Science Behind Movement and Healing

What I was experiencing wasn't just anecdotal—there's solid

science behind it. Research shows that physical movement can significantly aid in trauma recovery:

1. **Exercise and Neuroplasticity**: Regular physical activity promotes neuroplasticity, the brain's ability to form new neural connections. This is especially important for trauma survivors, whose brains may have been altered by their experiences. A study published in *Frontiers in Psychology* found that exercise can help the brain recover from trauma by enhancing neuroplasticity and supporting emotional regulation.

2. **Stress Reduction**: Physical activity helps reduce cortisol levels, the body's main stress hormone. A study in the *Journal of Clinical Psychiatry* revealed that individuals who engage in regular exercise have lower cortisol levels and report lower stress. This is crucial for trauma survivors, who often have elevated cortisol levels due to chronic stress.

3. **Mind-Body Practices**: Yoga, tai chi, and other mind-body practices have been shown to be particularly effective for trauma recovery. A study in *Traumatology* highlighted that trauma-sensitive yoga can significantly reduce PTSD symptoms and improve overall well-being by helping individuals reconnect with their bodies in a safe and controlled environment.

Finding My Own Path to Healing

As I continued my journey, I found that different forms of movement resonated with me in different ways. Some days, I craved the calm and stillness of yoga. On other days, I needed something more vigorous, like a run or a dance class, to shake off the restlessness that sometimes bubbled up inside me. Each form of movement offered something unique—a way to process emotions, release tension, or simply feel alive in my own skin again.

I also discovered the power of group activities. I joined a weekly dance class that was specifically geared toward trauma survivors. It wasn't about perfecting technique or learning choreography—it was about expressing ourselves through movement, in a space where we felt safe and supported. The rhythm of the music, the energy of the group, and the freedom to move without judgment created a sense of connection and healing that I hadn't found elsewhere.

How to Achieve the Thirteenth Law: Practical Steps

If you're looking to incorporate the thirteenth law of mental resilience, "Move to Heal," into your life, here are some practical steps that helped me:

1. **Start Small**: You don't need to dive into intense workouts right away. Start with simple movements that feel good to you, whether it's stretching, walking, or even just tossing a ball back and forth like I did with Steve. The goal is to reconnect with your body in a way that feels safe and manageable.

2. **Explore Different Activities**: Try out different forms of movement to see what resonates with you. Yoga, dance, tai chi, running—each offers its own benefits. Listen to your body and choose what feels right for you on any given day.

3. **Focus on How It Feels**: Rather than focusing on how you look or how well you're performing, pay attention to how the movement feels in your body. This can help you stay present and connected to the experience, rather than getting caught up in self-judgment.

4. **Join a Group**: If you feel comfortable, consider joining a group activity. Whether it's a class, a sports team, or a

walking group, the social aspect can enhance the healing benefits of movement by providing a sense of community and support.

5. **Be Patient**: Healing through movement is a process, and it's important to be patient with yourself. There will be days when it feels easy and days when it feels difficult. Honor where you are in your journey and trust that every small step is a step toward healing.

The thirteenth law of mental resilience, "Move to Heal," taught me that physical movement is not just about exercise—it's a powerful tool for healing from trauma. Through movement, I learned to release the tension stored in my body, reconnect with my emotions, and find a sense of safety and peace that I hadn't known was possible. Supported by scientific research and my own personal experiences, this law reminds us that our bodies hold the key to healing, and by moving, we can unlock the resilience within us.

Law 14

Resist the False Friends

"Substance abuse promises relief but delivers destruction."

This law speaks to the dangerous allure of substances like alcohol and drugs, especially for those grappling with the aftermath of trauma. These substances may seem like a quick escape, a way to numb the overwhelming pain, but they ultimately deepen the wounds, leading to greater despair and long-term harm. True healing requires confronting and processing trauma, not avoiding it through temporary and destructive means.

The Temptation to Numb the Pain

When trauma strikes, the emotional pain can be unbearable. Whether it's the constant replaying of a traumatic event, the relentless nightmares, or the anxiety that never seems to abate, the urge to escape it all can feel overwhelming. For many, substances like alcohol and drugs offer a seductive promise of relief—a brief respite from the relentless torment within. But this relief is an illusion, one that quickly fades, leaving behind a more profound sense of emptiness, shame, and despair.

The Downward Spiral of a Beloved Friend

I want to share the story of someone dear to me—let's call him David. David was the kind of person everyone loved to be around.

He had an infectious laugh, a gentle heart, and a talent for making those around him feel special. But beneath his warm exterior, David carried the heavy burden of unresolved trauma from his childhood. He never spoke much about it, but those close to him could see the pain in his eyes, the way he'd sometimes drift off in the middle of a conversation, lost in memories that were too painful to confront.

In his early twenties, David started to drink more frequently. It began innocently enough—a drink after work to unwind, a few beers with friends on the weekends. But as time went on, the drinking became more frequent and more intense. We all noticed the change, but it was hard to confront. After all, he seemed to have everything under control—he still made us laugh, still showed up for work, and still seemed like the David we all knew and loved. But behind closed doors, David was struggling. The alcohol wasn't just a way to unwind anymore; it was a way to escape. The memories of his childhood—memories he had spent years trying to suppress—began to surface with increasing intensity. The more he drank, the more those memories seemed to haunt him. And the more they haunted him, the more he drank to try and make them go away.

It wasn't long before alcohol wasn't enough. David started experimenting with drugs—first recreationally, then more seriously. He was chasing a numbness that alcohol alone could no longer provide. But instead of finding relief, he found himself sinking deeper into a pit of despair. The substances that promised to dull his pain only sharpened it, isolating him from the people who cared about him and pushing him further away from the life he once knew.

We all tried to reach out, to remind him of the person he was before the addiction took hold. But David was slipping away. He started missing work, avoiding friends, and withdrawing into himself. The vibrant, joyful person we had known was fading, replaced by someone we hardly recognized—someone whose life revolved around the next drink, the next hit, the next escape.

The Destructive Cycle of Substance Abuse

David's story is all too common. Research shows that individuals who experience trauma are significantly more likely to turn to substances as a form of self-medication. A study published in *The Journal of Clinical Psychiatry* found that people with PTSD are at a much higher risk of developing substance use disorders, as they seek ways to cope with the overwhelming symptoms of their trauma.

But this coping mechanism is a trap. The temporary relief that substances provide is quickly overshadowed by the long-term consequences. Substance abuse exacerbates the symptoms of trauma, leading to a vicious cycle where the individual becomes increasingly dependent on substances to function. The very tools they use to escape their pain end up intensifying it, isolating them further from the support they need to heal.

Historical data supports this understanding. For instance, among Vietnam War veterans, the rates of substance abuse were alarmingly high. Many veterans returned home with deep psychological scars and turned to alcohol and drugs to cope. According to the U.S. Department of Veterans Affairs, nearly 25% of Vietnam veterans struggle with substance use disorders. This statistic highlights the profound link between trauma and substance abuse, demonstrating how the false promise of relief can lead to a lifetime of struggle and pain.

The Path to True Healing: Confronting Trauma

Breaking free from the cycle of substance abuse is incredibly challenging, but it is possible. True healing requires immense courage—the courage to face the trauma that led to substance use, confront the pain head-on, and seek healthier ways to cope. Here's how to start:

1. **Acknowledge the Problem:** The first step is recognizing that substance use is not a solution but a symptom of deeper pain. It's important to acknowledge that while substances may offer temporary relief, they ultimately make the problem worse and hinder true healing.

2. **Seek Professional Help:** Recovery from both trauma and substance abuse often requires professional support. Therapists and counselors trained in trauma-informed care can help individuals navigate the complex emotions associated with trauma and develop healthier coping mechanisms.

3. **Build a Support System:** Surround yourself with people who understand and support your journey toward healing. This could include friends, family, support groups, or a combination of these. Having a strong support network can make a significant difference in your ability to resist the pull of substances and stay on the path to recovery.

4. **Practice Mindfulness and Self-Care:** Mindfulness practices, such as meditation and yoga, can help individuals stay grounded in the present moment and reduce the urge to numb their emotions. Self-care routines, including regular exercise, healthy eating, and sufficient sleep, are also crucial for maintaining physical and mental well-being during the recovery process.

5. **Confront the Trauma**: True healing requires facing the trauma that led to substance abuse in the first place. This might involve working through painful memories, processing emotions, and coming to terms with what happened. It's a difficult process, but one that is essential for reclaiming your life.

6. **Avoid Triggers**: Identify situations, people, or environments that trigger the urge to use substances and develop strategies to avoid or manage these triggers. This might involve making lifestyle changes, such as avoiding places where substances are readily available or finding new, healthy ways to cope with stress.

The fourteenth law of mental resilience, "Resist the False Friends," is a crucial reminder of the dangers of substance abuse, especially in the wake of trauma. David's story, like so many others, illustrates the devastating consequences of seeking refuge in alcohol and drugs. These substances may offer a temporary escape, but they ultimately deepen the pain, leading to a cycle of dependency and despair.

True healing requires confronting the trauma, not numbing it. By acknowledging the problem, seeking support, and taking active steps to face the trauma head-on, individuals can break free from the grip of substances and begin the journey toward true healing and resilience. It's a challenging path, but one that leads to a life of greater clarity, purpose, and peace—a life that David, like many others, deserved to find.

Law 15

Cultivate Gratitude

"Gratitude is not only the greatest of virtues but the parent of all the others." Cicero

"Gratitude is the antidote to despair." This law underscores the transformative power of gratitude in the face of life's challenges. When trauma and adversity cloud our minds, it's easy to focus on what's wrong, on the pain and the loss. But gratitude has the remarkable ability to shift our focus to what's right, to the small yet profound blessings that often go unnoticed. This simple act of appreciation can transform our perspective, reduce stress, and build resilience.

The Power of Gratitude: Shifting from Despair to Hope

Trauma has a way of pulling us into darkness. It magnifies our fears, amplifies our sorrows, and makes it difficult to see beyond the immediate pain. In such moments, the world can feel like a bleak and hopeless place. But even in the darkest times, there is light to be found—if we choose to see it. That light is gratitude.

Gratitude is not about ignoring the difficulties we face; it's about acknowledging the good that coexists with the challenges. It's about recognizing that, despite the hardships, there are still things to be thankful for. This shift in perspective doesn't magically erase the pain, but it does create space for healing. It reminds us that life is a complex tapestry of experiences, woven with both sorrow and joy.

The concept of gratitude in the face of life's hardships is powerfully reflected in *The Four Agreements* by Don Miguel Ruiz. One of the final teachings in the book is the idea that we should live each day as if it were our last, embracing life fully and expressing gratitude for every moment. This is akin to preparing for the "initiation of death"—a metaphorical death that symbolizes the shedding of old beliefs and fears, allowing us to live freely and fully in the present moment.

Ruiz writes about the importance of recognizing that everything in life is temporary and not truly ours to keep. The "angel of death" teaches us that everything—our possessions, relationships, and even our lives—can be taken away at any moment. Instead of living in fear of this loss, we are encouraged to surrender to it, to accept the impermanence of life, and to express gratitude for what we have, while we have it. This mindset is the key to cultivating a deep and lasting sense of peace and resilience.

Research on Gratitude: The Science Behind the Practice

The benefits of gratitude are not just philosophical; they are grounded in scientific research. Studies have consistently shown that practicing gratitude can have profound effects on our mental and physical health:

1. **Improved Mental Health**: A study published in the *Journal of Personality and Social Psychology* found that individuals who kept a gratitude journal, writing down things they were thankful for each day, experienced significant improvements in their mental health. They reported lower levels of depression and anxiety and a greater sense of overall well-being.

2. **Increased Resilience**: Research in the field of positive psychology has shown that gratitude increases resilience, particularly in the face of trauma. A study conducted by psychologists Robert Emmons and Michael McCullough found that individuals who practice gratitude are better able to cope with stress and recover from traumatic events. Gratitude helps shift focus from what's missing to what's present, fostering a mindset of abundance rather than scarcity.

3. **Better Physical Health**: Gratitude has also been linked to better physical health. A study published in *Psychosomatic Medicine* found that individuals who practiced gratitude had lower levels of the stress hormone cortisol, better immune function, and even lower blood pressure. These physical benefits contribute to an overall sense of well-being and vitality.

4. **Enhanced Relationships**: Gratitude has a powerful impact on relationships. Expressing appreciation for others strengthens bonds and fosters a sense of connection. A study in *Personal Relationships* found that partners who regularly expressed gratitude for each other felt more positive about their relationship and were more committed to staying together.

Viktor Frankl and the Power of Gratitude in the Holocaust

One of the most profound examples of the power of gratitude comes from Viktor Frankl, a Holocaust survivor and the author of *Man's Search for Meaning*. During his time in Nazi concentration camps, Frankl witnessed unimaginable horrors. Yet, even in the midst of such suffering, he found moments of grace—small acts of kindness, the beauty of a sunset, the warmth of a memory. These moments of gratitude became a lifeline, a way to maintain his humanity and his will to live.

Frankl's experience underscores the idea that gratitude is not dependent on external circumstances. Even in the darkest of times, there is something to be grateful for. By focusing on these small blessings, Frankl was able to find meaning and purpose in the midst of chaos and despair. His story is a powerful testament to the resilience that gratitude can cultivate, even in the most extreme conditions.

How to Cultivate Gratitude: Practical Steps

Gratitude is a practice that can be cultivated, even in the face of adversity. Here are some practical steps to help you integrate gratitude into your daily life:

1. **Start a Gratitude Journal**: Each day, write down three things you are grateful for. They don't have to be big or profound—simple things like a warm cup of coffee, a kind word from a friend, or the beauty of a sunrise are enough. Over time, this practice can help shift your focus from what's wrong to what's right in your life.

2. **Express Gratitude to Others**: Take the time to thank the people in your life who have made a difference, no matter how small. Whether it's a heartfelt note, a text message, or a verbal expression of thanks, acknowledging others fosters connection and spreads positivity.

3. **Practice Mindful Gratitude**: Throughout the day, pause and take a moment to appreciate your surroundings. Notice the little things—a blooming flower, the sound of birds chirping, the warmth of the sun on your skin. These mindful moments of gratitude can ground you in the present and remind you of the beauty in everyday life.

4. **Reframe Challenges**: When faced with difficulties, try to find something positive in the situation. This doesn't mean ignoring the challenges, but rather, looking for the silver

lining. For example, a tough work project might teach you new skills, or a disagreement with a friend might deepen your understanding of each other.

5. **Live Each Day as If It Were Your Last**: Inspired by *The Four Agreements*, remind yourself each morning that life is fleeting and precious. Approach each day to live fully, express love, and appreciate the moments you have. This mindset can shift your focus from fear and scarcity to gratitude and abundance.

The fifteenth law of mental resilience, "Cultivate Gratitude," teaches us that gratitude is more than just a positive emotion—it's a powerful tool for transforming our lives. By focusing on what's right rather than what's wrong, we can reduce stress, build resilience, and find peace even in adversity. Through the teachings of *The Four Agreements* and the experiences of individuals like Viktor Frankl, we see that gratitude is not just a practice for the good times, but a lifeline in the darkest moments.

Incorporating gratitude into our daily lives doesn't require grand gestures; it's about finding joy in the small things, appreciating the people around us, and living each day with the awareness that life is a precious gift. By doing so, we not only enhance our own well-being but also spread positivity to those around us, creating a ripple effect of resilience and hope.

Law 16

Know Your Triggers

"Until you make the unconscious conscious, it will direct your life and you will call it fate." Carl Jung

"Awareness is the first line of defense against the past." This law highlights the critical importance of understanding what triggers your trauma responses. By identifying these triggers, you can prepare for them and develop strategies to manage them effectively. In an age where anxiety and depression have become pervasive, particularly among younger generations, recognizing and understanding one's triggers is more essential than ever.

The Prevalence of Anxiety and Depression: A Growing Concern

Anxiety and depression are not just fleeting emotions; they have become defining mental health challenges of our time, particularly among young people. The statistics are alarming. A 2022 study of over 37,000 high school students in Wisconsin found that the prevalence of anxiety had risen from 34% in 2012 to 44% in 2018, with even higher rates among girls and LGBTQ teens. Similarly, a 2023 study of American college students revealed that 37% reported feeling anxious "always" or "most of the time," while another 31% felt this way "about half the time." This means only about one-third of college students experience anxiety less than half the time or never.

These figures suggest that a significant portion of young people are living in a near-constant state of distress. But why? What is driving this tidal wave of anxiety and depression? To understand this, we need to delve deeper into the nature of anxiety and its triggers.

The Biology of Fear and Anxiety

Fear is one of the most basic and essential emotions for survival across the animal kingdom. Our ancestors lived in a world full of predators, and those with the quickest responses to threats were more likely to survive and pass on their genes. Our brains are wired to trigger fear responses even before we fully process a threat, enabling us to react almost instantaneously. This is why you might jump out of the way of a car before you're even fully aware of its presence.

However, while fear is a response to an immediate threat, anxiety is triggered by the anticipation of a possible threat. It's healthy to be anxious in situations where danger might be lurking, as it keeps us alert and ready to react. But when this anxiety is triggered by ordinary, non-threatening events, it can spiral out of control, leading to a perpetual state of distress.

The Role of Social Threats

Our evolutionary history has also made us particularly sensitive to social threats. Human beings are social animals, and our survival has long depended on our ability to form strong social bonds. Being shunned or ostracized by the group was historically as dangerous as facing a physical predator. Today, this sensitivity to social threats manifests in the form of anxiety, especially in adolescents who are hyper-aware of their social standing.

The rise of social media has only exacerbated this problem. The constant comparison to others, fear of missing out (FOMO), and the pressure to present a perfect image online can trigger anxiety in young people, leading to a cycle of rumination, self-doubt, and distress.

Understanding and Managing Triggers

To manage anxiety and prevent it from spiraling into a disorder, it's crucial to identify and understand your triggers. Triggers are specific people, places, situations, or even thoughts that can set off a negative emotional response. These can be unique to each person, depending on their history, experiences, and personality.

For example, someone who has experienced bullying might feel anxious in crowded social settings where they feel scrutinized or judged. Another person who has endured a traumatic event might feel triggered by certain sounds, smells, or even weather conditions that remind them of that experience.

Recognizing these triggers is the first step in managing them. Once you know what sets off your anxiety, you can develop strategies to cope. This might involve avoiding certain situations, practicing relaxation techniques, or challenging the negative thoughts that arise when you're triggered.

Research on Anxiety and Triggers

Research supports the importance of understanding and managing triggers as a key component of mental health. Cognitive Behavioral Therapy (CBT), one of the most effective treatments for anxiety, focuses on helping individuals identify their triggers and develop strategies to cope with them. CBT teaches people to recognize distorted thinking patterns, such as catastrophizing or overgeneralizing, which often exacerbate anxiety. By addressing these thought patterns, individuals can reduce the intensity of their emotional responses to triggers.

A study published in *Behavior Research and Therapy* found that individuals who underwent CBT showed significant reductions in anxiety symptoms, particularly when they learned to identify and manage their triggers. The study emphasized that awareness of triggers is crucial for breaking the cycle of anxiety, as it allows individuals to anticipate their responses and implement coping mechanisms before their anxiety escalates.

The Anxiety of Social Exclusion

The concept of social anxiety isn't new; it has been recognized throughout history. One poignant example is the experience of "social death" in ancient societies. In ancient Rome, for instance, exile was considered one of the most severe punishments, often equated with a death sentence. Being cut off from the community meant losing one's identity, status, and support system, triggering profound anxiety and despair. This historical precedent illustrates how deeply rooted our fear of social exclusion is, and how it can manifest as anxiety in modern times.

How to Achieve the Sixteenth Law: Practical Steps

Understanding your triggers is essential to managing anxiety and building mental resilience. Here are some practical steps to help you achieve this:

1. **Keep a Trigger Journal**: Start by keeping a journal where you document situations that trigger your anxiety. Note the specific circumstances, your thoughts, physical sensations, and emotional responses. Over time, patterns will emerge, helping you identify your most common triggers.

2. **Practice Mindfulness**: Mindfulness practices, such as meditation and deep breathing, can help you stay grounded in the present moment. When you encounter a trigger, mindfulness can prevent you from being swept

away by the ensuing anxiety, allowing you to observe your thoughts and feelings without judgment.

3. **Develop Coping Strategies**: Once you've identified your triggers, develop specific strategies to manage them. This might include avoiding certain situations, challenging negative thoughts, or using relaxation techniques to calm your body's response.

4. **Seek Professional Help**: If your triggers are causing significant distress or interfering with your daily life, consider seeking help from a therapist. CBT and other therapeutic approaches can provide you with tools to manage your triggers effectively.

5. **Build a Support System**: Surround yourself with people who understand your struggles and can offer support. Talking about your triggers with trusted friends or family members can help reduce their power over you.

6. **Gradual Exposure**: In some cases, facing your triggers in a controlled and gradual manner can help desensitize you to them. This process, known as exposure therapy, is often used in treating phobias and anxiety disorders. It involves slowly and safely confronting your triggers until they no longer provoke a strong emotional response.

The sixteenth law of mental resilience, "Know Your Triggers," emphasizes the importance of self-awareness in managing anxiety and preventing it from spiraling out of control. In a world where anxiety and depression are increasingly common, particularly among young people, understanding your triggers is the first step toward building resilience.

By identifying what sets off your anxiety, you can prepare for these moments and develop strategies to manage them effectively. Supported by research and historical context, this law reminds us that awareness is the foundation of mental health. With the right tools and support, you can transform your triggers from sources of distress into opportunities for growth and healing.

Law 17

Reframe Your Thoughts

"It's not what happens to you, but how you react to it that matters." Epictetus

"Your thoughts are the architects of your reality." This law emphasizes the transformative power of your thoughts, particularly in the aftermath of trauma. Trauma survivors often find themselves trapped in negative thought patterns that reinforce feelings of hopelessness and despair. However, by learning to reframe these thoughts—such as turning "I'm broken" into "I'm healing"—you can change your mindset and empower your recovery journey.

The Power of Thought: Shaping Reality

Our thoughts shape the way we perceive the world and ourselves. For trauma survivors, negative thought patterns can become deeply entrenched, making it challenging to move forward. These thoughts might manifest as beliefs like "I'm worthless," "I'll never get better," or "I'm permanently damaged." Such beliefs can create a self-fulfilling prophecy, where the mind's narrative keeps the person stuck in a cycle of suffering.

However, the brain's ability to change—known as neuroplasticity—offers hope. This means that with intentional effort, we can reframe our thoughts and, in doing so, reshape our reality.

Reframing your thoughts involves taking control of the narrative you tell yourself. Instead of viewing yourself as a victim, you can start to see yourself as a survivor, someone who is actively healing and becoming stronger.

The Neuroscience Behind Reframing Thoughts

Cognitive neuroscience has shown that our thoughts significantly influence our mental and physical health. Negative thinking triggers the release of stress hormones like cortisol, leading to physical symptoms such as headaches, muscle tension, and a weakened immune system. Over time, chronic stress can contribute to mental health issues like anxiety and depression.

Conversely, positive thinking and reframing negative thoughts can have a powerful healing effect. Studies have shown that individuals who practice positive thinking experience lower stress levels, improved immune function, and greater overall well-being. Cognitive Behavioral Therapy (CBT), one of the most effective treatments for anxiety and depression, is based on the principle of reframing negative thoughts into more constructive ones.

A study published in the *Journal of Consulting and Clinical Psychology* highlighted the effectiveness of CBT in reducing symptoms of depression. The study found that patients who engaged in CBT showed significant improvements in mood and cognitive function, largely due to their ability to reframe negative thoughts and adopt a more positive outlook.

The Resilience of Malala Yousafzai: Reframing Tragedy into Triumph

One of the most inspiring examples of reframing thoughts comes from Malala Yousafzai, the young Pakistani activist who became a global symbol of resilience after surviving an attack by the Taliban.

Malala was only 15 years old when she was shot in the head by Taliban militants while riding a bus home from school. The attack was meant to silence her fight for girls' education, but instead, it strengthened her resolve and amplified her voice.

Reflecting on the attack, Malala once said, **"They thought that the bullets would silence us, but they failed. And then, out of that silence came thousands of voices."** Despite the trauma she endured, Malala chose to reframe her experience. Rather than succumbing to fear or anger, she viewed the attack as a catalyst for even greater advocacy. She refused to see herself as a victim; instead, she embraced her role as a survivor and an advocate for the millions of girls around the world who are denied an education.

Malala's ability to reframe her thoughts transformed her reality. Instead of being defined by her trauma, she became the youngest-ever Nobel Peace Prize laureate, a powerful voice for education, and a symbol of hope and resilience. As she put it, **"I tell my story not because it is unique, but because it is the story of many girls."**

Her story demonstrates how reframing negative thoughts can lead to empowerment and positive change, even in the face of unimaginable adversity.

How to Achieve the Seventeenth Law: Practical Steps

Reframing your thoughts is a powerful tool for transforming your mindset and empowering your recovery. Here are some practical steps to help you achieve this:

1. **Identify Negative Thought Patterns**: Start by becoming aware of your negative thinking patterns. Notice the thoughts that arise when you're feeling stressed, anxious, or depressed. Are there recurring themes or beliefs that keep coming up?

2. **Challenge Your Thoughts**: Once you've identified a negative thought, challenge its validity. Ask yourself: Is this thought based on facts, or is it a distorted perception? What evidence do you have to support or refute this thought? This process of questioning helps to weaken the hold that negative thoughts have on you.

3. **Reframe the Thought**: After challenging the negative thought, reframe it in a more positive or realistic light. For example, if you find yourself thinking, "I'm a failure," try reframing it to, "I'm learning and growing from my experiences." The goal is to shift your perspective from one of self-criticism to one of self-compassion and growth.

4. **Practice Gratitude**: Gratitude is a powerful antidote to negative thinking. By focusing on what you're thankful for, you can counterbalance negative thoughts and cultivate a more positive outlook. Consider keeping a gratitude journal where you write down three things you're grateful for each day.

5. **Use Affirmations**: Positive affirmations are statements that reinforce healthy beliefs about yourself. Repeating affirmations such as "I am strong," "I am healing," or "I am capable of overcoming challenges" can help reprogram your mind and replace negative thought patterns with empowering ones.

6. **Seek Professional Support**: If you find it difficult to reframe your thoughts on your own, consider seeking help from a therapist. CBT and other therapeutic approaches can provide you with the tools and guidance needed to effectively change your thinking patterns.

7. **Mindfulness Meditation**: Mindfulness meditation can help you become more aware of your thoughts and create space between your thoughts and your reactions. This

awareness allows you to observe your thoughts without judgment and choose how to respond to them, rather than reacting automatically.

8. **Surround Yourself with Positivity**: The people you spend time with and the media you consume can greatly influence your thoughts. Surround yourself with positive influences—friends, mentors, books, and podcasts that uplift and inspire you.

The seventeenth law of mental resilience, "Reframe Your Thoughts," is a powerful reminder that our thoughts shape our reality. Trauma can distort your thinking, leading to negative beliefs that perpetuate suffering. However, by consciously reframing these thoughts, you can change your mindset, empower your recovery, and create a life filled with possibility and hope.

Through the lens of cognitive neuroscience and the inspiring example of Malala Yousafzai, we see that while we may not always have control over our circumstances, we do have control over how we interpret and respond to them. By practicing the art of reframing, you can transform your inner narrative from one of despair to one of hope and resilience, setting the stage for true healing and growth. As Malala wisely said, **"We realize the importance of our voices only when we are silenced."**

Law 18

Release Resentment

"Holding onto anger is like drinking poison and expecting the other person to die." – Buddha

Forgiveness is the ultimate act of self-liberation. Holding onto anger and resentment can poison your spirit. Forgiveness isn't about excusing what happened; it's about freeing yourself from the burden of bitterness.

Understanding Resentment and Its Impact

Imagine waking up one morning, full of energy and optimism for the day ahead. But then, a heated argument with your spouse over breakfast drains your energy, leaving you emotionally exhausted. The weight of anger and resentment lingers, casting a dark shadow over your entire day. This is the destructive power of resentment.

Every day, we start with a finite amount of mental, emotional, and physical energy. How we manage this energy determines our ability to live fulfilling lives. When we allow resentment to consume us, it depletes our energy reserves, leaving us with little capacity for joy, creativity, or meaningful connections with others.

Resentment and Perception: Our perception of the world is deeply influenced by the emotions we carry. When we harbor resentment, everything around us seems tainted. The weather, the people we encounter, and even the simplest tasks become sources of irritation. In contrast, when we release resentment, the world appears brighter, and we regain the ability to see the beauty in everyday life.

The Emotional Wounds of Resentment

Resentment can be likened to a festering wound on the mind. Just as an infected wound on the skin causes physical pain, emotional wounds infected with resentment cause mental and emotional suffering. These wounds can become so deeply ingrained that they distort our perception of reality, leading us to believe that such pain is normal.

Imagine a world where everyone's mind is covered in these emotional wounds, where the pain is so prevalent that it's considered normal. People would distance themselves from one another, avoiding close connections to protect themselves from further pain. This is the reality for many who carry unresolved resentment—isolated, mistrustful, and burdened by a constant undercurrent of anger.

The Power of Forgiveness

Forgiveness is the antidote to resentment. It's not about condoning the wrongs done to us but about liberating ourselves from the emotional poison that resentment brings. By forgiving, we reclaim our energy, our peace, and our ability to live fully in the present.

Research supports the transformative power of forgiveness. Studies have shown that individuals who practice forgiveness experience lower levels of stress, anxiety, and depression. Forgiveness has also been linked to improved physical health, including lower blood pressure and a stronger immune system. By releasing resentment, we not only heal our minds but also strengthen our bodies.

The Process of Forgiveness

Forgiveness is a journey, not a one-time event. It begins with acknowledging the pain and resentment we carry and understanding its impact on our lives. We must then make a conscious decision to forgive, not because the other person deserves it, but because we deserve peace.

Self-Forgiveness: An essential part of this process is self-forgiveness. Often, the hardest person to forgive is ourselves. We may blame ourselves for allowing the hurt to happen, for our reactions, or for holding onto the pain for so long. But true healing begins when we forgive ourselves and embrace self-compassion.

A Historical Example: Nelson Mandela's Path to Forgiveness

Nelson Mandela's life offers a powerful example of the liberating power of forgiveness. After spending 27 years in prison for his fight against apartheid in South Africa, Mandela emerged not with a heart full of bitterness but with a commitment to reconciliation. He understood that forgiveness was not just for the oppressors but also for himself and his nation.

Mandela famously said, **"Resentment is like drinking poison and then hoping it will kill your enemies."** By choosing forgiveness, Mandela helped heal a divided nation and became a global symbol of peace and reconciliation.

Practical Steps to Release Resentment

1. **Acknowledge the Pain:** Begin by recognizing the resentment you hold and how it affects your life.

2. **Reflect on the Impact:** Consider how holding onto resentment drains your energy and prevents you from living fully.

3. **Choose Forgiveness:** Make a conscious decision to forgive, not for the sake of others, but for your own well-being.

4. **Practice Self-Forgiveness:** Release the blame you place on yourself and embrace self-compassion.

5. **Seek Support:** If the burden of resentment feels too heavy to bear alone, seek support from a therapist, counselor, or trusted friend.

6. **Cultivate Gratitude:** Shift your focus from the wrongs done to you to the blessings in your life. Gratitude can help dissolve resentment and restore peace.

Releasing resentment is an act of self-liberation. It frees us from the chains of bitterness and allows us to reclaim our energy, our peace, and our ability to live fully in the present. By choosing forgiveness, we take the first step towards healing our minds and hearts, paving the way for a life filled with joy, connection, and true resilience.

The 48 Laws of Mental Power

Law 19

Establish Your
Boundaries

"Daring to set boundaries is about having the courage to love ourselves, even when we risk disappointing others." — Brené Brown

Boundaries are the lines that protect your peace. For trauma survivors, setting clear boundaries is crucial for safeguarding their well-being and preventing further harm. Boundaries help create a protective barrier around your mental, emotional, and physical space, ensuring that only positive and supportive influences are allowed in. This law emphasizes the importance of establishing and maintaining boundaries as a means of self-preservation and healing.

Trauma often leaves individuals vulnerable and more susceptible to further hurt. Without firm boundaries, it becomes easy for others to overstep, leading to repeated patterns of emotional distress and harm. Establishing boundaries is not about isolation; it's about creating a safe space where healing can occur. It's about knowing where you end and others begin and having the strength to enforce those lines.

The Role of Boundaries in Healing

Research shows that people who establish and maintain clear boundaries are more resilient and better equipped to handle stress. A study published in the *Journal of Counseling Psychology* found that individuals who assertively communicate their boundaries report higher levels of self-esteem and lower levels of stress and depression. This is particularly important for trauma survivors, who may struggle with feelings of guilt, shame, or worthlessness that make it difficult to stand up for themselves.

In one of the more poignant studies, researchers examined the impact of boundary-setting on individuals with a history of abuse. The study revealed that those who learned to establish firm boundaries experienced significant improvements in their emotional and psychological well-being. They reported fewer instances of anxiety, depression, and PTSD symptoms, compared to those who did not set boundaries.

Historical Instance: Rosa Parks and the Power of Boundaries

One of the most powerful examples of establishing boundaries can be seen in the story of Rosa Parks. On December 1, 1955, Parks refused to give up her seat to a white passenger on a segregated bus in Montgomery, Alabama. This act of defiance was not just a stand against racial injustice; it was a profound assertion of her boundaries. By refusing to move, Parks drew a line that said, "Enough." Her boundary-setting became a catalyst for the Civil Rights Movement, showing how powerful and transformative it can be to assert one's dignity and self-respect.

Parks later said, "I was not tired physically... No, the only tired I was, was tired of giving in." Her boundary-setting was an act of self-liberation, and it resonated across the nation, empowering others to stand up for their rights.

Achieving This Law

1. **Identify Your Boundaries**: The first step in establishing boundaries is identifying what they are. Consider what makes you feel uncomfortable or unsafe and where you need to draw the line to protect your well-being. This could be in relationships, at work, or even with family.

2. **Communicate Clearly**: Once you've identified your boundaries, communicate them clearly and assertively. You don't have to justify your boundaries to anyone. It's enough to state them and expect them to be respected.

3. **Enforce Your Boundaries**: It's not enough to just set boundaries; you must also be willing to enforce them. This means being prepared to walk away from situations or people who do not respect your limits.

4. **Self-Care and Reflection**: Regularly check in with yourself to ensure your boundaries are still serving you. Boundaries can evolve, and it's important to adjust them as necessary to reflect your current needs.

5. **Seek Support**: If you find it difficult to set or enforce boundaries, consider seeking support from a therapist or counselor. They can help you develop the skills needed to protect your peace and well-being.

Boundaries are essential for anyone, but especially for those who have experienced trauma. They protect your peace, ensure your safety, and empower you to live a life free from the shadows of the past. Remember, establishing boundaries is an act of self-respect and self-care. It is a powerful way to reclaim your life and ensure that your environment supports your healing journey.

Law 20

Reconnect with the Earth

"Look deep into nature, and then you will understand everything better."— Albert Einstein

Nature is not merely a backdrop to our lives; it is a profound healer that asks nothing in return. In a world increasingly dominated by technology and urbanization, we often find ourselves disconnected from the very essence that grounds us—the Earth. Yet, countless studies have shown that spending time in nature can calm the nervous system, reduce stress, and foster a deep sense of connection and well-being. This 20th law of mental power— reconnecting with the Earth—is about reclaiming that lost bond and allowing nature to heal and nourish our weary souls.

The Healing Power of Nature

Consider the simple act of walking barefoot on grass, known as "grounding" or "earthing." Research has shown that this practice can reduce inflammation, improve sleep, and enhance overall well-being by reconnecting us with the Earth's natural electric charge. A study published in the JOURNAL OF ENVIRONMENTAL AND PUBLIC HEALTH in 2012 found that grounding the body to the Earth alters the electrical activity in the brain, leading to reduced stress and improved mood.

Similarly, spending time in forests, a practice the Japanese call SHINRIN-YOKU or "forest bathing," has been shown to lower blood pressure, reduce cortisol levels, and boost the immune system. A 2010 study from Nippon Medical School in Tokyo demonstrated that a few hours in the forest could significantly increase the number of natural killer cells, which are crucial for fighting off infections and cancer.

These benefits are not just psychological but deeply physiological, showing how nature's rhythms can bring our own bodies back into balance. The Earth, with its vast forests, flowing rivers, and open skies, offers us a sanctuary—a place where we can shed the stress of modern life and reconnect with our most authentic selves.

How to Reconnect with the Earth

Reconnecting with the Earth doesn't require grand gestures; it can be as simple as spending time outdoors each day. Here's how to achieve this reconnection:

1. **Daily Nature Time**: Whether it's a walk in the park, a hike in the mountains, or simply sitting in your backyard, make it a daily practice to spend time in nature. Let the sights, sounds, and smells of the natural world envelop you.
2. **Grounding Exercises**: Practice grounding by walking barefoot on natural surfaces like grass, sand, or soil. This simple act can have profound effects on your well-being, helping you feel more centered and connected.
3. **Forest Bathing**: Engage in SHINRIN-YOKU by immersing yourself in a forest or wooded area. The act of simply being in nature, breathing in the fresh air, and observing the natural world around you can reduce stress and rejuvenate your spirit.
4. **Gardening**: Tending to a garden, no matter how small, can be a deeply grounding experience. The act of nurturing

plants, feeling the soil in your hands, and witnessing the cycle of growth can foster a deep connection to the Earth.

5. **Mindful Observation**: Take time to observe the natural world with mindfulness. Watch the clouds drift, listen to the birds sing, or feel the breeze on your skin. This practice of mindful observation can help you develop a greater appreciation for the beauty and healing power of nature.

The Tree as a Metaphor for Healing

Imagine a young tree that has been injured—it grows around that injury, adapting and continuing its upward climb. As the tree matures, the wound becomes a small part of its overall structure, adding character and beauty to its form. This tree is a powerful metaphor for how we, as human beings, can grow around our own wounds and traumas. The tree doesn't deny its injury; it incorporates it into its being, using the experience to shape its unique character.

Similarly, trauma can leave deep scars on our psyche, but nature teaches us that these scars don't have to define us. By reconnecting with the Earth, we can find the strength to grow around our wounds, integrating them into the fabric of our lives in a way that adds depth and resilience to our character.

The Science Behind Nature's Healing

Studies have consistently shown that nature has a profound impact on our mental and physical health. A landmark study published in NATURE in 2019 found that spending just 120 minutes a week in nature is associated with good health and well-being. The study revealed that individuals who spent at least two hours in nature per week were more likely to report good health and psychological well-being compared to those who did not.

Furthermore, the practice of forest bathing has been shown to reduce the levels of the stress hormone cortisol, which is linked to anxiety and depression. A 2011 study in ENVIRONMENTAL HEALTH AND PREVENTIVE MEDICINE reported that participants who spent time in a forest environment had lower cortisol levels, lower blood pressure, and a greater sense of calm than those who spent time in an urban environment.

Nature is a healer that requires nothing from us but our presence. By reconnecting with the Earth, we not only soothe our nervous systems and reduce stress, but we also find a deeper sense of connection and grounding. This reconnection allows us to heal from the wounds of the past, just as a tree grows around its injuries, using them to shape its unique beauty. In a world that often pulls us away from our natural roots, the 20th law of mental power reminds us to return to the Earth, to find solace and strength in its embrace, and to allow its healing power to restore our peace and well-being.

Law 21

Rediscover Joy

"The purpose of life is to live it, to taste experience to the utmost, to reach out eagerly and without fear for a newer and richer experience."— *Eleanor Roosevelt*

Life often throws challenges our way that leaves us feeling like we're merely surviving, moving through our days without truly living. Trauma and hardship can strip us of our joy, leaving us disconnected from the activities and passions that once brought us happiness. But rediscovering joy, particularly through hobbies and activities that ignite your spirit, is essential for healing and reclaiming your life.

Imagine Sarah, a dedicated nurse who spent years caring for others but had forgotten how to care for herself. The long hours, the emotional toll of the job, and the weight of her responsibilities had left her feeling empty. She moved through her days like a robot, performing her duties but feeling no real connection to life. It wasn't until her therapist suggested she reconnect with an old hobby that things began to change.

Sarah had always loved painting. As a child, she would spend hours with her brushes and colors, losing herself in the creation of vibrant worlds on canvas. But as she grew older, life's demands took over, and the brushes were packed away, forgotten in a dusty corner of her closet.

One evening, after a particularly draining day at the hospital, Sarah found herself pulling out the old box of paints. Hesitant at first, she dipped her brush into the rich colors, and as she began to paint, something inside her shifted. The stress of the day melted away with each stroke, replaced by a sense of calm and satisfaction. For the first time in years, she felt connected to something deeper, something joyful.

The Science Behind Joy and Hobbies

Research supports what Sarah experienced. Engaging in hobbies and creative activities can have a profound impact on mental health. Studies have shown that people who regularly engage in hobbies report higher levels of happiness and lower levels of stress and depression. A 2016 study published in the *Journal of Positive Psychology* found that individuals who spent time on creative activities felt more enthusiastic and had a higher sense of well-being the next day.

Furthermore, engaging in hobbies can help rewire the brain. Neuroscientific research suggests that creative activities like painting, knitting, or playing a musical instrument stimulate the brain's reward centers. This not only provides immediate pleasure but also fosters long-term resilience by reinforcing positive neural pathways.

Healing Through Joy: The Importance of Reconnecting

Trauma often leaves us vulnerable and disconnected from the things that once brought us happiness. It's easy to fall into the trap of just getting through the day, especially when past experiences have made joy feel out of reach. But rediscovering joy is not just a luxury; it's a necessity for healing.

Sarah's journey back to painting was more than just a return to an old hobby; it was a reclamation of her sense of self. Each time she picked up the brush, she was reminded that life is not just about enduring hardships; it's also about finding moments of beauty and peace. Painting became her way of reconnecting with herself, of telling the world that she was more than her job, more than her responsibilities. She was a person who deserved joy.

How to Rediscover Joy

1. **Reflect on Past Passions:** Take a moment to think about what activities used to bring you joy. Was it dancing, writing, gardening, or perhaps playing a sport? These past passions can serve as a gateway to rediscovering your joy.
2. **Start Small:** If it's been a while since you engaged in a hobby, start small. Dedicate just 10-15 minutes a day to doing something you love. Gradually increase the time as you become more comfortable.
3. **Experiment:** Don't be afraid to try new things. Sometimes, discovering a new hobby can be just as fulfilling as returning to an old one. Take a class, join a group, or simply experiment at home.
4. **Prioritize Joy:** Make time for hobbies and joyful activities, even if it means rearranging your schedule. Joy is not a luxury; it's an essential part of a healthy, fulfilling life.
5. **Share Your Joy:** Connect with others who share your interests. Join a community or group where you can share your hobby and connect with like-minded individuals.

Rediscovering joy through hobbies is about more than just passing the time—it's about healing, reconnecting with yourself, and finding fulfillment in life's small pleasures. As Sarah found with her painting, these activities can be a powerful tool in your journey toward wholeness.

Law 22

Arm Yourself with Knowledge

"Knowledge is power." — *Sir Francis Bacon*

Knowledge turns fear into understanding. Understanding is not just a matter of grasping abstract concepts; it is a transformative tool that can turn fear and confusion into clarity and control. When you understand the science of trauma, as Bessel van der Kolk explores in *The Body Keeps the Score*, you begin to see that trauma is not just an event but a physiological response that affects both mind and body. By arming yourself with this knowledge, you gain the power to take control of your healing, rather than being at the mercy of your past experiences. Knowledge is not just a remedy; it is a powerful weapon in overcoming the effects of trauma.

I have a friend named Becky, who once seemed to have it all together—a successful career, a loving family, and a bright future. But beneath the surface, she carried the invisible scars of childhood trauma. For years, Becky struggled with anxiety, panic attacks, and a deep sense of unworthiness. Despite her outward success, she felt broken inside, haunted by memories she couldn't fully understand or control.

Becky's turning point came when she stumbled upon *The Body Keeps the Score* by Bessel van der Kolk. It was as if a light had been switched on in a dark room. For the first time, she began to understand that her symptoms were not signs of weakness or failure but were rooted in her body's response to trauma. She learned that trauma changes the way the brain functions, altering how it processes emotions, memories, and even bodily sensations.

One of the key insights Becky gained was how trauma can recalibrate the brain's alarm system, leading to hypervigilance and a constant sense of danger. She realized that her panic attacks were her brain's way of trying to protect her, even though the threat was long gone. This knowledge transformed her perspective—her panic was no longer a terrifying mystery, but a challenge she could address.

Research supports the profound impact that understanding trauma can have on recovery. For instance, studies in neuroscience have shown that trauma physically alters brain structures, particularly the amygdala (the brain's alarm system), the hippocampus (responsible for memory), and the prefrontal cortex (involved in decision-making and self-regulation). These changes explain why traumatized individuals often feel stuck in a cycle of fear and why they struggle to regulate their emotions.

Moreover, developmental psychopathology, a field studying how adverse experiences affect brain development, has revealed that trauma can disrupt normal emotional and cognitive growth. This disruption often manifests in difficulties with learning, relationships, and self-regulation later in life. By understanding these effects, individuals can begin to address the root causes of their struggles rather than merely treating the symptoms.

Turning Knowledge into Power

Arming yourself with knowledge is not just about reading books or attending therapy sessions; it's about applying that understanding to your life. Becky began to use mindfulness practices, such as deep breathing and body scanning, to reconnect with her body and calm her overactive alarm system. She also started cognitive-behavioral therapy (CBT) to reframe her traumatic memories and see them as part of her past, not her present.

Becky's journey was not easy, but with each step, she gained more control over her mind and body. The more she understood about how trauma affected her, the less power it had over her. She learned that recovery is not about forgetting the past but about integrating it into the broader narrative of her life.

How to Achieve Law 22: Arm Yourself with Knowledge

1. **Educate Yourself**: Start by reading books, such as *The Body Keeps the Score*, that explain the science of trauma. Understanding how trauma affects the brain and body will demystify your experiences and give you a framework for healing.
2. **Seek Professional Guidance**: Work with a therapist trained in trauma-informed care. Techniques such as Eye Movement Desensitization and Reprocessing (EMDR) or somatic experiencing can help you process traumatic memories and reconnect with your body.
3. **Practice Mindfulness**: Incorporate mindfulness practices into your daily routine. These can help you stay grounded in the present moment and reduce the impact of traumatic triggers.
4. **Join Support Groups**: Connect with others who have experienced similar traumas. Sharing your experiences and hearing others' stories can provide comfort, reduce isolation, and foster a sense of community.
5. **Apply Knowledge to Your Life**: Use your understanding of trauma to change your thought patterns and behaviors. For example, recognizing that a panic attack is a physiological response rather than a personal failure can help you manage it more effectively.

Arming yourself with knowledge is the first step toward reclaiming your life from the shadows of trauma. Like Becky, you can transform fear into understanding and take control of your healing journey. Knowledge is not just a tool; it's a shield and a sword, empowering you to face your past and move forward with strength and resilience.

Law 23

Express Without Words

"I found I could say things with color and shapes that I couldn't say any other way—things I had no words for." - Georgia O'Keeffe

Creativity is the voice that speaks when words fail. Sometimes, words are not enough to express the depth of your emotions. Creative outlets like art, music, or dance can help you process and release feelings that are difficult to verbalize.

In a world where words often dominate our expressions, there are moments when they simply fall short. The pain of a lost loved one, the confusion of a life-altering decision, or the overwhelming joy of a new beginning—these emotions run so deep that language alone cannot capture them. This is where creativity steps in, offering a way to express what words cannot.

The Power of Creative Expression

When my friend Jenna lost her father, she was paralyzed by grief. Talking about it only seemed to amplify her pain, and no amount of comforting words could soothe her. One day, she found herself at an art supply store, inexplicably drawn to a blank canvas. Without any formal training, Jenna began to paint. The brush became an extension of her heart, each stroke a release of the emotions she could not articulate. The colors on the canvas danced between dark and light, capturing her grief and the love she still held for her father. This painting, she later told me, became her voice when words failed.

Creative expression, whether through art, music, dance, or writing, offers a powerful way to process emotions. Research supports this. A study published in *The American Journal of Public Health* found that creative activities can significantly reduce stress, anxiety, and depression while enhancing well-being and quality of life. The study highlighted that when people engage in creative activities, they experience a sense of fulfillment and accomplishment that contributes to their emotional health.

Creativity and Trauma

Trauma often leaves us feeling disconnected from ourselves and the world around us. The brain, in its attempt to protect us, can block access to certain memories and emotions, making them difficult to process through traditional means. However, creative expression can bypass these blocks, allowing us to explore and release emotions in a non-threatening way.

Consider the work of Dr. Bessel van der Kolk, a leading expert in trauma treatment and author of *The Body Keeps the Score*. Van der Kolk emphasizes that trauma impacts the brain in such a way that traditional talk therapy alone may not be sufficient. Instead, he advocates for using creative outlets, such as art or movement, to help trauma survivors reconnect with their emotions and begin the healing process. Neuroimaging studies support this approach, showing that activities like drawing, dancing, or playing music activate different parts of the brain than those engaged during verbal communication. This can help trauma survivors process their experiences on a deeper level.

A Story of Healing Through Dance

Another friend, Marcus, found his voice through dance. After surviving a traumatic car accident, Marcus struggled with anxiety and nightmares. Therapy sessions helped, but he still felt something was missing. One evening, he wandered into a dance studio where a group was practicing improvisational dance. The freedom of movement, the rhythm of the music, and the connection with others in the room offered Marcus a release he hadn't felt in years. Dance became his sanctuary—a place where he could express his fears, frustrations, and eventually, his healing. Through dance, Marcus was able to reframe his trauma, transforming it from a source of pain into a powerful narrative of resilience.

Achieving the 23rd Law

To fully embrace Law 23, it's essential to explore different creative outlets and find the one that resonates with you. Start by asking yourself what form of expression feels most natural. Is it painting, sculpting, writing poetry, playing an instrument, or perhaps dancing? Once you've identified your creative outlet, make it a regular part of your routine. Dedicate time each day or week to engage in this activity, allowing yourself to express whatever emotions arise without judgment or expectation.

For those who find it challenging to start, consider taking a class or joining a group. The social aspect can provide encouragement and inspiration. Remember, creativity is not about perfection; it's about expression. Your art doesn't have to be gallery-worthy, your music doesn't need to be concert-ready, and your dance doesn't need to be stage-perfect. What matters is that it reflects your emotions and helps you process them.

The Science Behind Creativity and Emotion

Scientific studies have shown that engaging in creative activities can have profound effects on mental health. For example, a 2010 study published in the *Journal of the American Art Therapy Association* found that 45 minutes of art-making significantly reduced levels of cortisol, a stress hormone, in the participants. Another study from *Frontiers in Psychology* highlighted that music therapy can improve emotional regulation and reduce symptoms of PTSD in trauma survivors. These findings underscore the idea that creativity is not just a hobby but a powerful tool for emotional expression and healing.

In a world that often prioritizes words, remember that creativity offers a different, equally valuable form of communication. Whether through art, music, dance, or any other medium, creative expression allows you to process and release emotions that words cannot capture. By embracing this law, you give yourself the freedom to explore the depths of your emotions and find healing in the most unexpected places. Just like Jenna and Marcus, you too can discover that creativity is the voice that speaks when words fail.

Law 24

Test Your Limits

*"Life begins at the end of your comfort zone." –
Neale Donald Walsch*

Strength is Found in the Stretch Beyond Comfort. Healing and growth are intrinsically linked, and neither can occur without pushing beyond the boundaries of what feels comfortable. The human capacity for resilience and adaptation is remarkable, but it requires us to venture into the unknown, to test our limits, and to embrace the discomfort that comes with this journey.

The Science Behind Testing Your Limits

Neuroplasticity: The Brain's Ability to Adapt

One of the most compelling pieces of evidence supporting the idea of testing your limits comes from research on **neuroplasticity**. Neuroplasticity refers to the brain's ability to reorganize itself by forming new neural connections throughout life. This ability allows the brain to adapt to new challenges, learn new skills, and recover from injuries.

In a landmark study published in NATURE by Dr. Eleanor Maguire and colleagues in 2000, the brains of London taxi drivers were examined to see how their intensive navigation experience affected brain structure. The study found that the hippocampus—a region of the brain associated with spatial memory—was significantly larger in taxi drivers compared to non-drivers. This enlargement was directly correlated with the number of years spent driving, suggesting that the brain had physically adapted to the demands of their job. This research illustrates that when we push our cognitive limits, our brain responds by developing new capacities.

The Yerkes-Dodson Law: The Optimal Level of Challenge

The **Yerkes-Dodson Law**, first established in 1908, provides another scientific basis for testing your limits. This principle suggests that there is an optimal level of arousal (or challenge) that leads to peak performance. Too little challenge results in boredom, while too much can lead to stress and anxiety. However, when the level of challenge is just right—slightly above what feels comfortable—it leads to heightened focus, engagement, and ultimately, better performance.

A study published in the JOURNAL OF PERSONALITY AND SOCIAL PSYCHOLOGY in 2010 by Andrew Elliot and Holly Thrash explored this phenomenon further. They found that individuals who are slightly outside their comfort zones experience increased motivation and better performance, particularly when the challenges align with their personal goals. This supports the idea that pushing beyond comfort is crucial for growth.

The Growth Mindset: Embracing Challenges

Dr. Carol Dweck's research on the **growth mindset** offers critical insights into why testing our limits is essential for personal development. Dweck, a psychologist at Stanford University, found that individuals who believe their abilities can be developed (a growth mindset) are more likely to embrace challenges and persist in the face of setbacks.

In her studies, Dweck observed that students with a growth mindset were more willing to tackle difficult tasks and learn from their mistakes, while those with a fixed mindset tended to avoid challenges to protect their self-esteem. Over time, those with a growth mindset showed significant improvements in their academic performance and overall resilience. This research highlights the importance of adopting a mindset that welcomes challenges as opportunities for growth.

The Impact of Testing Limits in Childhood and Adolescence

Developmental Psychology: The Role of Risky Play

During childhood and adolescence, the opportunity to test limits is critical for healthy development. **Developmental psychology** shows that engaging in risky play—such as climbing, exploring, and testing physical boundaries—helps children learn to manage fear, develop problem-solving skills, and build confidence.

A study by Dr. Ellen Sandseter, published in EVOLUTIONARY PSYCHOLOGY in 2011, found that children who engage in risky play tend to have better emotional regulation and lower levels of anxiety as they grow older. Sandseter's research suggests that these experiences teach children to navigate challenges and uncertainties, which are essential skills for adulthood.

However, modern societal trends have increasingly restricted children's opportunities for risky play. **Dr. Peter Gray**, a psychologist and researcher, has written extensively on how the decline of free play and increased adult supervision have contributed to rising levels of anxiety and depression among young people. His research emphasizes that children need the freedom to test their limits to develop resilience and independence.

Strategies for Testing Your Limits

1. **Start Small**: The process of testing your limits doesn't have to be overwhelming. Begin with small, manageable challenges that push you just slightly out of your comfort zone. Over time, these small steps can lead to significant growth as you build confidence and resilience.
2. **Set Incremental Goals**: Breaking down larger goals into smaller, achievable milestones can make the process less daunting. Each small victory builds momentum and encourages you to keep pushing further.
3. **Embrace Failure as Feedback**: Viewing failure as a natural part of the learning process can help reduce the fear of taking on challenges. Research shows that individuals who see failure as feedback rather than a setback are more likely to persist in their efforts and ultimately succeed.
4. **Seek Supportive Environments**: Surrounding yourself with a supportive community can provide the encouragement and motivation needed to continue pushing your limits. Whether it's through mentorship, peer support, or collaborative environments, having others who believe in your potential can make a significant difference.
5. **Reflect and Adjust**: Regularly reflecting on your progress and making necessary adjustments is key to continued growth. This reflective practice allows you to learn from your experiences and refine your approach to future challenges.

The Broader Implications: Testing Limits in Adulthood

Testing your limits is not just for children and adolescents; it remains crucial throughout adulthood. **Research in organizational psychology** indicates that employees who are encouraged to step outside their comfort zones and take on new challenges tend to be more engaged, productive, and satisfied with their work. A study published in THE ACADEMY OF MANAGEMENT JOURNAL in 2015 by Dr. Teresa Amabile and her colleagues found that employees who were given challenging assignments that stretched their capabilities reported higher levels of job satisfaction and professional growth.

Moreover, **physical challenges** in adulthood, such as participating in endurance sports or taking on new physical activities, have been shown to improve mental health and cognitive function. A 2013 study published in THE JOURNAL OF AGING AND PHYSICAL ACTIVITY demonstrated that older adults who engaged in regular physical challenges experienced improvements in memory, attention, and overall cognitive function. This underscores the importance of continuing to push physical limits as a means of maintaining mental and physical health.

The science is clear: pushing beyond your comfort zone is essential for growth, whether it's in the brain's capacity to adapt, the development of resilience in childhood, or the pursuit of personal and professional goals in adulthood. By testing your limits, you not only discover new strengths but also cultivate the resilience needed to navigate life's challenges.

Remember, growth is not a linear process, and the journey of testing your limits will come with its share of setbacks. But each step you take beyond what feels comfortable brings you closer to realizing your full potential. As you continue to test your limits, you'll find that what once seemed impossible becomes not only achievable but also a source of strength and pride.

Law 25

Trust the Process

"Patience and perseverance have a magical effect before which difficulties disappear and obstacles vanish." — John Quincy Adams

Patience is the Quiet Power that Sustains the Journey. Healing from trauma is a journey marked by peaks and valleys, progress, and setbacks. It's easy to feel discouraged when the path to recovery seems long and winding, but it's essential to remember that healing is not a race—it's a process. Patience is the quiet power that sustains this journey, allowing us to trust that every step, no matter how small, is moving us closer to recovery.

The Science of Patience in Healing

Neurobiology of Trauma: Understanding the Internal Process

Trauma fundamentally alters the brain's functioning. Research by Dr. Bessel van der Kolk, a pioneering psychiatrist in the field of trauma, has shown that traumatic experiences can cause lasting changes in the brain, particularly in areas responsible for memory, emotion regulation, and self-perception. The amygdala, the brain's alarm system, becomes hyperactive, while the prefrontal cortex, responsible for rational thought and decision-making, often shuts down during trauma, leading to a state of heightened arousal and reactivity.

Van der Kolk's research, detailed in his book THE BODY KEEPS THE SCORE, emphasizes the importance of working with the body to heal trauma. He argues that because trauma is stored in the body, the process of recovery must also engage the body, not just the mind. This understanding underscores the importance of patience in healing, as the brain and body require time to reorganize and integrate traumatic experiences.

The Role of the Parasympathetic Nervous System

The **parasympathetic nervous system (PNS)** plays a crucial role in the body's recovery from trauma. It is responsible for the "rest and digest" functions, which counteract the "fight or flight" responses triggered by the sympathetic nervous system during traumatic events. Activating the PNS through practices like deep breathing, mindfulness, and yoga can help calm the body and mind, reducing the chronic stress and hyperarousal associated with trauma.

A study published in FRONTIERS IN PSYCHOLOGY in 2016 demonstrated that regular mindfulness meditation significantly reduces symptoms of PTSD by enhancing the functioning of the PNS. This finding highlights the importance of cultivating patience and trust in the healing process, as these practices require consistent effort over time to yield results.

Patience and the Process of Renegotiation

Understanding Trauma Reenactment

Trauma often leads to reenactment, where individuals unconsciously replay aspects of their traumatic experiences in their current lives. Sigmund Freud referred to this as "repetition compulsion," an attempt by the unconscious mind to resolve what remains unresolved. However, reenactment often fails to bring resolution because it keeps the trauma external, rather than processing it internally.

Carl Jung also noted that what remains unconscious does not dissolve but reemerges in our lives as fate. This is why trusting the process of healing is so crucial. By turning inward and patiently working through the emotions and sensations associated with trauma, individuals can begin to dismantle the patterns that drive reenactment. This process requires patience, as it involves accessing deeply buried memories and emotions, which can be overwhelming if not approached with care.

The Felt Sense and Healing

The concept of the **felt sense**, introduced by psychotherapist Eugene Gendlin, is key to understanding how trauma can be renegotiated. The felt sense is the body's internal awareness of a situation, an internal cue that tells us how we truly feel about an experience. By paying attention to the felt sense, individuals can begin to understand where their blockages are and how to move through them at a pace that feels safe.

Gendlin's research, published in FOCUSING (1978), showed that people who could connect with their felt sense and process their emotions through this bodily awareness were more successful in therapy. This highlights the importance of patience in the healing process—moving too quickly can overwhelm the nervous system, while moving too slowly may result in stagnation. Trusting the process means allowing the experience to unfold naturally, at a pace that supports integration and healing.

Strategies for Cultivating Patience in the Healing Process

1. **Practice Mindfulness and Meditation**: Mindfulness practices help ground you in the present moment, reducing anxiety about the future and regrets about the past. Regular meditation has been shown to lower cortisol levels and increase parasympathetic activity, promoting relaxation and emotional regulation.
2. **Engage in Somatic Practices**: Trauma is stored in the body, so engaging in somatic practices like yoga, tai chi, or dance can help release stored tension and trauma. These practices encourage you to move at your own pace, fostering a sense of safety and control.
3. **Develop a Supportive Network**: Surrounding yourself with a supportive community—whether through therapy, support groups, or trusted friends—can provide encouragement and validation throughout your healing journey. Sharing your experiences with others who understand can alleviate feelings of isolation and promote patience.
4. **Set Small, Achievable Goals**: Break down your healing journey into small, manageable steps. Celebrate each milestone, no matter how small, as progress. This approach reduces feelings of being overwhelmed and fosters a sense of accomplishment, reinforcing your trust in the process.
5. **Journal Your Progress**: Keeping a journal can help you track your progress and reflect on your journey. Writing about your experiences allows you to process emotions and see how far you've come, which can strengthen your resolve and patience.

The Broader Implications: Trusting the Process in Life

The Role of Patience in Personal and Professional Growth

The concept of trusting the process extends beyond trauma healing and into all areas of life. In personal and professional growth, patience is often the difference between success and failure. The **Yerkes-Dodson Law** reminds us that optimal performance is achieved when we are challenged but not overwhelmed. Patience allows us to navigate challenges without rushing, giving us the time needed to develop the skills and resilience required for long-term success.

A study published in HARVARD BUSINESS REVIEW in 2015 found that leaders who practiced patience were more effective in decision-making, had better relationships with their teams, and were more likely to achieve long-term success. The study emphasized that patience is not passive; it involves active engagement and a deep understanding of the complexities of any given situation.

Trusting the process is not about passivity or resignation; it's about recognizing that true healing and growth take time. The science of trauma recovery, from the neurobiology of stress to the role of the felt sense, shows us that patience is a critical component of the journey. By cultivating patience, we allow ourselves the time and space needed to heal deeply and completely.

Every step, no matter how small, is a victory. Every moment of patience strengthens your ability to navigate the complexities of healing and growth. Trust that the process, with all its ups and downs, is moving you toward recovery and transformation.

Law 26

Stay Engaged

"We are all broken, that's how the light gets in." — *Ernest Hemingway*

Isolation is the enemy; connection is the cure. Trauma often leads to isolation, but staying connected with others is crucial. Engaging with supportive communities or loved ones can provide the connection needed to heal.

Isolation is a silent enemy that often accompanies trauma, wrapping individuals in a cocoon of solitude that deepens the wounds rather than heals them. When people experience trauma, the natural instinct might be to withdraw from the world, to retreat into the safety of isolation where they believe they can avoid further harm. However, this instinct, while understandable, can lead to further emotional and psychological damage. The 26th law of mental power emphasizes the importance of staying engaged with others as a crucial element of healing.

The Cost of Isolation: A Scientific Perspective

Research has shown that isolation has profound negative effects on mental and physical health. A study published in the *American Journal of Public Health* found that social isolation can increase the risk of premature death by up to 29%. This is comparable to other well-known risk factors such as smoking, obesity, and lack of physical activity. The study also highlighted that the effects of isolation are particularly severe for individuals who have experienced trauma, as they are already vulnerable to psychological distress.

One of the reasons isolation is so harmful is because it can exacerbate feelings of depression and anxiety. When people cut themselves off from others, they lose the opportunity to experience the positive reinforcement and emotional support that social connections provide. This lack of support can make it difficult to process and recover from traumatic experiences.

Furthermore, isolation can impair cognitive function. A study conducted by the University of Chicago found that social isolation can lead to cognitive decline, particularly in areas related to memory and executive function. The study revealed that people who are isolated are more likely to experience memory loss and have difficulty making decisions, both of which can hinder the healing process after trauma.

The Power of Connection: Healing Through Engagement

Staying connected with others is not just about having a social life; it's about creating a support system that can help individuals navigate the complexities of trauma recovery. Research has consistently shown that strong social connections are one of the most important factors in promoting mental health and well-being.

In one study published in the *Journal of Traumatic Stress*, researchers found that individuals who maintained strong social ties after experiencing trauma were more likely to recover and exhibit resilience. These connections provided emotional support, practical assistance, and a sense of belonging that helped them process their experiences and move forward.

Engaging with others can also provide a sense of purpose and meaning. Trauma often leaves individuals feeling disoriented and disconnected from their previous sense of self. By staying engaged with loved ones, communities, or supportive groups, individuals can begin to rebuild their identities and find new meaning in their lives.

Achieving Connection: Practical Steps

To stay engaged after trauma, it's important to take proactive steps to maintain and strengthen social connections. Here are some strategies:

1. **Join a Support Group:** Support groups provide a safe space for individuals to share their experiences and connect with others who have gone through similar situations. These groups can offer validation, understanding, and encouragement, which are crucial for healing.
2. **Reconnect with Loved Ones:** Trauma can strain relationships, but it's important to reach out to family and friends who can offer support. Even if it feels difficult, taking small steps to reconnect can make a big difference.
3. **Engage in Community Activities:** Participating in community events or volunteering can provide a sense of purpose and help individuals feel connected to something larger than themselves. These activities also offer opportunities to meet new people and build new relationships.
4. **Seek Professional Help:** A therapist or counselor can provide guidance on how to rebuild social connections after trauma. They can also help individuals navigate the emotional challenges that come with staying engaged.
5. **Practice Mindfulness:** Mindfulness techniques, such as meditation or yoga, can help individuals stay present and connected to their emotions. This awareness can make it easier to reach out to others and engage in meaningful interactions.

Isolation may seem like a safe haven after trauma, but it often deepens the wounds rather than heals them. By staying engaged with others, individuals can create a support system that fosters healing and resilience. The 26th law of mental power reminds us that connection is not just a luxury; it is a vital component of recovery. By reaching out to loved ones, joining supportive communities, and staying active in the world, individuals can find the strength to heal and thrive after trauma.

Law 27

Learn to Say No

"You have to decide what your highest priorities are and have the courage—pleasantly, smilingly, non-apologetically—to say 'no' to other things. And the way to do that is by having a bigger 'yes' burning inside."— Stephen Covey

Protect Your Energy by Mastering the Art of Refusal. In a world that constantly demands our attention, energy, and resources, learning to say "no" becomes not just an act of self-preservation but a crucial strategy for maintaining mental health and well-being. This law emphasizes the importance of setting boundaries to protect yourself from the draining effects of overcommitment and stress. Prioritizing your well-being over pleasing others is not an act of selfishness; rather, it is an essential practice for sustaining your mental, emotional, and physical health.

The Power of Boundaries

Boundaries are the invisible lines that define what is acceptable in our interactions and relationships. They serve as a shield against the demands and expectations that others may impose on us, helping to preserve our energy and mental clarity. Without clear boundaries, we risk becoming overwhelmed by the needs and desires of others, leading to burnout, stress, and diminished well-being.

Research in psychology consistently shows that people who set and maintain strong boundaries experience lower levels of stress and higher levels of satisfaction in their lives. A study published in the *Journal of Personality and Social Psychology* found that individuals who can assertively say "no" to unnecessary demands are more likely to have better mental health and experience less anxiety and depression.

The Cost of People-Pleasing

The inability to say "no" often stems from a desire to please others, to be liked, or to avoid conflict. However, this people-pleasing behavior can have significant negative consequences. A study from the *American Psychological Association* highlights that chronic people-pleasers are more prone to stress-related illnesses, such as cardiovascular disease and autoimmune disorders. This is because constantly prioritizing others' needs over your own can lead to chronic stress, which takes a toll on both mental and physical health.

Moreover, when we say "yes" to everything, we dilute our effectiveness. Our energy becomes scattered, and our ability to focus on what truly matters is compromised. This is often referred to as the "tyranny of the urgent," where we spend so much time responding to immediate demands that we neglect long-term goals and personal growth.

The Science Behind Saying No

The act of saying "no" is closely linked to the concept of self-control and executive function, which are governed by the prefrontal cortex of the brain. This area is responsible for decision-making, impulse control, and goal-oriented behavior. Studies in neuroscience have shown that the ability to say "no" is a key indicator of self-regulation and overall mental resilience.

One groundbreaking study conducted by researchers at Stanford University, known as the "Marshmallow Test," revealed that children who could delay gratification (i.e., say "no" to immediate temptations) were more likely to succeed in various areas of life, including academic achievement and emotional stability. This ability to resist immediate demands and prioritize long-term goals is a skill that can be developed and honed over time.

The Power of Saying No in the Workplace

Dr. Lisa Martin, a 42-year-old highly respected cardiologist at a major metropolitan hospital, was known for her dedication to her patients and her willingness to take on additional responsibilities. Over the years, Dr. Martin developed a reputation as the "go-to" person for any extra tasks or coverage needed in the hospital. However, this reputation came at a significant cost to her mental and physical well-being.

Dr. Martin's workload increased steadily, with her frequently working 60-70 hours a week. Her responsibilities expanded to include not only patient care but also administrative duties, teaching responsibilities, and participation in various hospital committees. Despite her exhaustion, Dr. Martin found it difficult to refuse requests from colleagues and supervisors. She felt a strong need to please everyone and maintain her reputation as a reliable and hard-working doctor.

By the time Dr. Martin reached her early forties, she began experiencing symptoms of burnout. These included chronic fatigue, insomnia, and a significant decrease in job satisfaction. She found herself becoming increasingly irritable and less compassionate toward her patients. Her performance started to decline, and she began making minor errors that she would have never made before. Dr. Martin's personal life also suffered, as she had little time or energy left for her family and friends.

Recognizing that her current trajectory was unsustainable, Dr. Martin sought help from a therapist who specialized in workplace stress and burnout.

Intervention: Learning to Say No

During therapy, Dr. Martin learned about the importance of setting boundaries and protecting her energy by saying "no" to additional demands that did not align with her priorities. She began to understand that her inability to say "no" was rooted in a fear of disappointing others and a desire to be perceived as indispensable. However, this mindset was contributing to her burnout and diminishing her effectiveness as a doctor.

The therapist introduced Dr. Martin to several practical strategies for learning to say "no" effectively:

1. **Identifying Priorities**: Dr. Martin was encouraged to clarify her professional and personal priorities. She realized that providing high-quality patient care, maintaining her health, and spending time with her family were her top priorities. Administrative duties and extra committee work, while important, were not as critical.

2. **Assertiveness Training**: Dr. Martin practiced assertive communication techniques with her therapist. This involved role-playing scenarios in which she would decline additional responsibilities politely but firmly. For example, when asked to take on an extra shift, she learned to say, "I'm currently managing a full workload and need to prioritize my existing responsibilities. I won't be able to cover the shift this time."

3. **The Pause Technique**: Dr. Martin learned to use a "pause" technique before responding to requests. When approached with a new task, she would take a moment to consider her current workload and how the request aligned with her priorities before giving an answer. This helped her avoid impulsively agreeing to tasks she didn't have the capacity to handle.

4. **Offering Alternatives**: To ease the discomfort of saying "no," Dr. Martin was taught to offer alternatives when appropriate. For example, if she was asked to join another

committee, she might respond with, "I'm unable to join this committee due to my current commitments, but I can suggest a colleague who may be interested."

Outcome

Over several months, Dr. Martin began implementing these strategies in her daily work life. Initially, she found it challenging to say "no," but with practice, she became more comfortable asserting her boundaries. She noticed several positive changes:

- **Reduced Workload**: By saying "no" to additional non-essential tasks, Dr. Martin was able to reduce her workload significantly. This allowed her to focus more on patient care and spend more time with her family.
- **Improved Mental Health**: With a more manageable workload, Dr. Martin's symptoms of burnout began to subside. She experienced less fatigue, started sleeping better, and regained her enthusiasm for her work.
- **Enhanced Job Performance**: With more time and energy to dedicate to her core responsibilities, Dr. Martin's job performance improved. She was able to provide better care for her patients and felt more fulfilled in her role as a doctor.
- **Stronger Professional Relationships**: Interestingly, learning to say "no" did not damage Dr. Martin's relationships with her colleagues as she had feared. Instead, her colleagues respected her for setting boundaries and were more mindful of her time. This led to more efficient and focused collaboration.

Scientific Corroboration

Dr. Martin's case is supported by a growing body of research that emphasizes the importance of boundary-setting and refusal in maintaining mental health and preventing burnout. A study published in the *Journal of Occupational Health Psychology* found that employees who set clear boundaries between work and personal life experienced lower levels of stress and higher job satisfaction. Another study in the *Journal of Behavioral Medicine* demonstrated that individuals who regularly practice assertiveness, including saying "no," reported better mental health outcomes, including reduced anxiety and depression.

Moreover, research has shown that learning to say "no" is particularly important in high-stress professions like healthcare. A study in the *British Medical Journal* highlighted that doctors who set limits on their work hours and responsibilities were less likely to experience burnout and were more likely to deliver high-quality patient care.

Dr. Lisa Martin's journey illustrates the critical importance of learning to say "no" as a means of protecting one's mental and physical health. By mastering the art of refusal and setting boundaries, she was able to regain control over her life, improve her well-being, and enhance her professional effectiveness. Her case serves as a powerful reminder that saying "no" is not a weakness but a strength that allows us to prioritize what truly matters and maintain our health and happiness.

Law 28

Celebrate the Small Wins

"Success is the sum of small efforts, repeated day in and day out."— Robert Collier

In the journey toward personal growth and mental fortitude, it is easy to overlook the significance of small achievements. Yet, it is these minor victories that lay the foundation for monumental progress. Celebrating small wins is not just a form of self-encouragement but a critical strategy for building momentum, reinforcing positive behaviors, and maintaining motivation over the long haul.

Research in psychology and behavioral science consistently highlights the importance of recognizing and celebrating small wins. A study conducted by Teresa Amabile and Steven Kramer at Harvard Business School, published in their book *The Progress Principle*, reveals that the single most important factor in boosting motivation, creativity, and positive emotions at work is making progress in meaningful work. Their study involved analyzing nearly 12,000 diary entries from 238 employees across seven companies, leading to the conclusion that small, daily progress is a more powerful motivator than even financial incentives.

Amabile and Kramer's research underscores that acknowledging minor victories triggers the brain's reward system, releasing dopamine, a neurotransmitter associated with pleasure and motivation. This creates a positive feedback loop, where the satisfaction of achieving a small goal drive further action and effort. In essence, each small win builds upon the last, gradually leading to more significant accomplishments.

Historical Insights: The Power of Incremental Progress

History is replete with examples of how small, consistent efforts can lead to remarkable achievements. Consider the story of the Allied forces during World War II. The D-Day invasion of Normandy on June 6, 1944, was a massive and complex operation, but it was the result of years of smaller victories. Each minor success— securing supply lines, gathering intelligence, training troops—was a step forward in the eventual liberation of Europe. The leaders of the Allied forces understood that each small win was crucial to the ultimate victory, and they celebrated these milestones to maintain morale and momentum.

In a more personal example, the great artist Michelangelo famously said, "If people knew how hard I worked to get my mastery, it wouldn't seem so wonderful at all." His masterpieces, including the Sistine Chapel, were not the result of sudden inspiration but of painstaking, incremental progress. Each brushstroke and each day of labor contributed to the final, breathtaking result. Michelangelo's journey was a testament to the power of small wins in achieving greatness.

The Science of Habit Formation

The concept of celebrating small wins is also deeply intertwined with the science of habit formation. James Clear, in his bestselling book *Atomic Habits*, explains that habits are formed through a cycle of cue, craving, response, and reward. When you set a small goal and achieve it, the satisfaction serves as a reward, reinforcing the behavior and making it more likely to be repeated. Over time, these small habits compound, leading to substantial changes in behavior and life outcomes.

Clear emphasizes that the key to lasting change is not in setting grand, sweeping goals, but in focusing on small, manageable tasks that can be accomplished daily. By celebrating these small wins, you provide the necessary reinforcement for these new behaviors to stick, gradually building a foundation for larger successes.

Practical Application: How to Celebrate Small Wins

1. **Set Clear, Achievable Goals**: Break down larger goals into smaller, manageable tasks. For instance, if you aim to write a book, start by setting a goal to write 200 words a day. Each day you meet that target, recognize it as a victory.
2. **Keep a Progress Journal**: Document your progress daily or weekly. Writing down your achievements, no matter how minor, helps you see the accumulation of small wins over time, reinforcing your sense of accomplishment.
3. **Reward Yourself**: After completing a small goal, reward yourself with something meaningful. It could be as simple as taking a short break, enjoying a favorite snack, or spending time on a hobby. These rewards help cement the positive feeling associated with the achievement.
4. **Share Your Wins**: Sharing your achievements with friends, family, or a supportive community can amplify the positive effects of small wins. Social reinforcement can enhance motivation and keep you accountable.
5. **Reflect on Your Progress**: Periodically take the time to look back at how far you've come. This reflection can help you appreciate the cumulative effect of your small wins and encourage you to keep going.

Conclusion: Building a Foundation for Success

Celebrating small wins is not just a motivational tool but a strategic approach to achieving long-term success. By recognizing and rewarding incremental progress, you build momentum, reinforce positive behaviors, and maintain motivation even in the face of challenges. Whether you are working on a personal project, advancing in your career, or striving for mental well-being, remember that progress is built on the foundation of small victories. Each step forward, no matter how small, is a crucial part of the journey toward your ultimate goals.

Victor O. Carl

Law 29

Embrace Your Unique Path

"Comparison is the thief of joy." — *Theodore Roosevelt*

Comparisons are thieves; your journey is yours alone. In a world saturated with social media and constant exposure to the lives of others, it's easy to fall into the trap of comparison. Whether it's scrolling through curated images of others' successes, witnessing their achievements, or even observing their healing processes, the urge to compare your journey to theirs can be overwhelming. However, such comparisons are not just unproductive; they can be detrimental to your mental health and personal growth. This law emphasizes the importance of embracing your unique path, recognizing that everyone's journey is different, and focusing on your own progress without letting the experiences of others cloud your vision.

The Danger of Comparison

Comparison, as the old adage goes, is the thief of joy. Research by psychologist Dr. Sherry Turkle from the Massachusetts Institute of Technology (MIT) has shown that constant exposure to others' lives through social media can lead to increased feelings of inadequacy and depression. This phenomenon is particularly prevalent in younger generations, where the pressure to conform to societal standards or achieve what others have seemingly accomplished can create a relentless cycle of self-doubt and dissatisfaction.

155

A study conducted by the University of Houston found a direct link between social media use and depressive symptoms, largely due to the habit of social comparison. The more individuals compared themselves to others online, the more likely they were to experience depressive thoughts. This is because when you compare yourself to others, you are often comparing your entire self to someone else's highlight reel—a distorted reality that rarely shows the full picture of their struggles and setbacks.

The Uniqueness of Your Path

Understanding that your journey is uniquely yours is crucial to maintaining mental well-being and achieving personal growth. No two people have the same life experiences, challenges, or resources. Even in the realm of healing from trauma or pursuing personal development, each individual's path is distinct.

Dr. Carol Dweck's research on the growth mindset emphasizes that progress is not about how you compare to others but how you improve over time. When you embrace your unique path, you focus on your growth, measuring yourself against where you were yesterday rather than where someone else is today. This shift in perspective fosters resilience, motivation, and a sense of accomplishment.

For instance, studies in neuroplasticity, the brain's ability to reorganize itself by forming new neural connections, have shown that personal progress is deeply individual. The rate at which someone heals from trauma or learns new skills depends on various factors, including genetic predisposition, environmental support, and personal effort. Comparing your progress to others ignores these variables and can lead to unnecessary frustration.

The Role of Self-Compassion

To embrace your unique path fully, practicing self-compassion is essential. Dr. Kristin Neff, a pioneer in the field of self-compassion research, highlights that self-compassion involves treating yourself with the same kindness and understanding that you would offer to a friend in times of struggle. This approach helps reduce the negative impact of comparison by shifting the focus from what you lack to what you can nurture within yourself.

Self-compassion has been linked to lower levels of anxiety and depression, higher life satisfaction, and greater emotional resilience. By acknowledging that your path is unique and that setbacks are a natural part of growth, you allow yourself the grace to move forward at your own pace, free from the burden of unrealistic comparisons.

Real-World Examples

Consider the story of J.K. Rowling, who faced numerous rejections before finally getting her manuscript for *Harry Potter* accepted. Had she compared her journey to that of other successful authors, she might have given up. Instead, she embraced her unique path, understanding that her journey was different but no less valuable.

Similarly, Oprah Winfrey's journey was filled with personal struggles and setbacks. Rather than comparing her path to others, she focused on her own growth and development, which ultimately led to her incredible success.

Achieving Law 29: Practical Steps

1. **Limit Social Media Exposure:** Reduce time spent on platforms that encourage comparison. Instead, engage in activities that promote self-reflection and personal growth.
2. **Set Personal Goals:** Focus on setting and achieving your own goals based on your values and aspirations, not on what others are doing. Celebrate small victories and milestones that reflect your progress.

3. **Practice Gratitude:** Regularly reflect on what you have accomplished and what you are grateful for. This practice shifts your attention away from what others have that you don't, fostering a more positive mindset.
4. **Mindful Reflection:** Engage in mindfulness practices that help you stay present and grounded in your own journey. This can include meditation, journaling, or simply taking time to reflect on your experiences without judgment.
5. **Seek Supportive Communities:** Surround yourself with people who understand and respect your unique journey. Supportive friends, mentors, or therapists can provide encouragement and perspective, helping you stay focused on your path.
6. **Affirm Your Progress:** Regularly affirm the steps you've taken on your journey, no matter how small they may seem. Acknowledge that progress is not always linear and that every step forward is valuable.
7. **Practice Self-Compassion:** Understand that it's okay to move at your own pace. Practice self-compassion by acknowledging that everyone has different strengths and challenges. Being kind to yourself is essential in maintaining a positive mindset.

Your journey is yours alone, and it is uniquely valuable. By embracing your path, you give yourself the freedom to grow and heal at your own pace. Remember, the only person you should compare yourself to is who you were yesterday. By focusing on your progress and staying true to your own journey, you will find fulfillment and success that is uniquely yours.

Law 30

Master the Breath

"Feelings come and go like clouds in a windy sky. Conscious breathing is my anchor." — *Thich Nhat Hanh*

Breath control is the key to controlling the mind; breathing exercises can calm your mind and body, reducing anxiety and stress. Mastering the breath is a powerful tool in managing trauma responses.

Breath control is the key to mastering the mind. This law, grounded in ancient wisdom and modern science, emphasizes the profound link between our breath and mental state. Mastering breath can calm the mind, reduce anxiety, and allow us to navigate trauma responses more effectively. In today's fast-paced world, the ability to control our breath and thus control our emotional state is more important than ever.

The Science of Breath Control

Breath, though often taken for granted, is one of the most powerful tools we have for self-regulation. Studies in neuroscience and psychology have demonstrated that the breath has a direct impact on the brain and the body's autonomic nervous system. Specifically, it influences the balance between the sympathetic nervous system, responsible for the fight-or-flight response, and the parasympathetic nervous system, which promotes rest and relaxation.

One of the critical components here is the **vagus nerve**, which connects the brain to many internal organs, including the heart, lungs, and digestive system. The vagus nerve plays a crucial role in the parasympathetic nervous system. When activated through deep, slow breathing, it helps to lower heart rate, reduce blood pressure, and calm the mind. **80% of the vagus nerve's fibers are afferent, meaning they send signals from the body to the brain**, allowing us to control mental states through physical processes like breathing.

Research published in the *Journal of Clinical Psychology* in 2016 found that individuals who practiced deep breathing techniques regularly experienced significant reductions in stress levels, anxiety, and depressive symptoms. This is a scientific validation of what ancient traditions in India and China have long known: control the breath, and you control the mind.

Historical and Cultural Significance

For centuries, cultures across the world have utilized breath control as a central element in spiritual and healing practices. In India, **pranayama** (breath control) is a cornerstone of yoga, designed to channel energy, calm the mind, and harmonize the body. Tai Chi and Qi Gong in China also emphasize breathing as a way to cultivate inner peace and physical health. In religious practices, rhythmic breathing during chanting or prayer serves to calm both body and soul.

Despite the deep-rooted traditions of these non-Western approaches, modern psychiatry has, until recently, focused largely on pharmaceutical interventions to manage anxiety, trauma, and stress. However, a growing body of research now points to breath control as a highly effective, non-invasive technique for emotional regulation. Studies from the National Institutes of Health (NIH) have shown that **10 weeks of yoga and breathwork** significantly reduced the symptoms of PTSD in individuals who had not responded to medication or traditional therapy.

How Trauma Affects the Breath

Trauma often leaves individuals in a heightened state of arousal. The fight-or-flight response becomes chronically activated, leading to shallow, rapid breathing that reinforces feelings of anxiety and panic. For people with PTSD, the body's natural alarm system is always on, causing hypervigilance and an inability to relax. This chronic over-activation leads to a host of physical symptoms like increased heart rate, insomnia, and gastrointestinal issues.

One of the most effective ways to counteract this is through conscious, controlled breathing. **Slow, deep breaths signal to the brain that the threat has passed**, engaging the parasympathetic nervous system and shutting down the fight-or-flight response. Research from the University of Pittsburgh demonstrated that deep diaphragmatic breathing not only reduced symptoms of anxiety but also improved overall cognitive function by increasing oxygen flow to the brain.

The Practical Application of Breath Mastery

How can you master your breath to control your mind and emotions? Here are practical steps to implement Law 30 in your daily life:

1. **Diaphragmatic Breathing (Belly Breathing):**

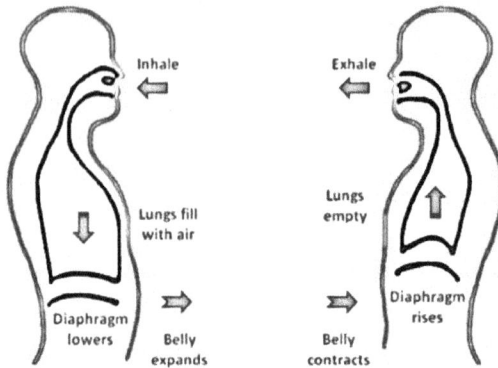

- o Place one hand on your chest and the other on your abdomen.
- o Take a deep breath through your nose, ensuring that your abdomen (not your chest) rises.
- o Exhale slowly through your mouth, feeling your abdomen fall.
- o Repeat this process for 5-10 minutes daily, focusing on slow, deep, and intentional breaths.

Research shows that diaphragmatic breathing reduces cortisol levels, the hormone responsible for stress, leading to a calmer and more focused mind.

2. **4-7-8 Breathing Technique:**

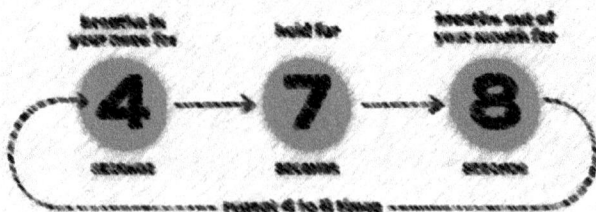

- o Inhale through your nose for a count of 4.
- o Hold your breath for a count of 7.
- o Exhale slowly through your mouth for a count of 8.

o Repeat for four cycles. This method is known for calming the nervous system and reducing anxiety.

The 4-7-8 technique was popularized by Dr. Andrew Weil and has been found effective for managing stress, particularly before sleep.

3. **Box Breathing (Square Breathing):**

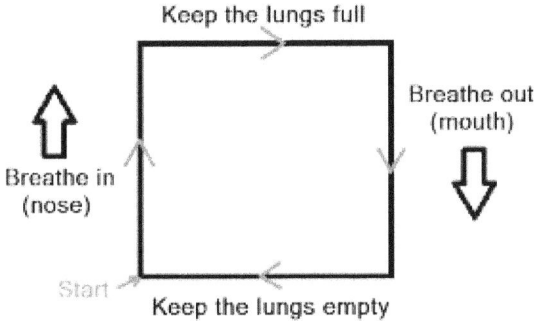

Keep the lungs full

Breathe out (mouth)

Breathe in (nose)

Start

Keep the lungs empty

o Inhale for a count of 4.
o Hold your breath for a count of 4.
o Exhale for a count of 4.
o Hold again for a count of 4.
o Repeat for several cycles.

This method is used by Navy SEALs to remain calm under pressure and increase focus. A study published in the *Journal of Sports Science & Medicine* found that box breathing significantly improved cognitive function and emotional resilience in high-stress environments.

4. **Alternate Nostril Breathing (Nadi Shodhana):**
o Close your right nostril with your thumb and inhale deeply through your left nostril.
o Close your left nostril and exhale through your right.
o Inhale through the right nostril, then close it and exhale through the left.
o Continue alternating for several minutes.

This technique balances the brain's hemispheres and is particularly effective for reducing anxiety and promoting mental clarity.

Case Study: Transforming Trauma Through Breath Mastery

Meet **Alex Thompson**, a 35-year-old veteran who returned from active duty with severe PTSD. Alex struggled with hyperarousal, flashbacks, and emotional numbness, severely impacting his personal and professional life. Traditional treatments, including cognitive-behavioral therapy (CBT) and medication, provided limited relief.

Intervention: Integrating Breath Control

Determined to find alternative solutions, Alex enrolled in a holistic trauma recovery program that emphasized breath control alongside conventional therapies.

1. Initial Assessment

Alex's therapist conducted a comprehensive assessment, identifying his primary symptoms: chronic anxiety, insomnia, and difficulty managing emotions. Recognizing the role of the autonomic nervous system in his condition, the therapist introduced diaphragmatic breathing and mindfulness meditation as complementary strategies.

2. Implementation of Breath Techniques

- **Diaphragmatic Breathing:** Alex began practicing belly breathing twice daily, gradually increasing the duration as he became more comfortable.
- **Box Breathing:** Before bed, Alex used box breathing to calm his mind and prepare for restful sleep.

- **Mindful Breathing Meditation:** Alex incorporated 15 minutes of mindful breathing each morning to set a positive tone for the day.

3. Progress and Outcomes

After eight weeks, Alex reported significant improvements:

- **Reduced Anxiety:** Episodes of panic and hyperarousal decreased in frequency and intensity.
- **Improved Sleep Quality:** Alex experienced fewer disturbances and felt more rested upon waking.
- **Enhanced Emotional Regulation:** He became more adept at managing his emotions, leading to better relationships and increased job performance.

4. Scientific Corroboration

Alex's progress mirrors findings from studies such as those published in the *Journal of Clinical Psychology*, which demonstrate that integrating breath control with traditional therapies enhances overall treatment efficacy for PTSD patients.

Integrating Breath Mastery into Daily Life

To fully embrace **Law 30: Master the Breath**, it's essential to incorporate breath control into your daily routine. Here's how to make it a seamless part of your life:

1. Start Small

Begin with short sessions of diaphragmatic breathing or box breathing. Even five minutes a day can set the foundation for deeper practice.

2. Create Triggers for Practice

Associate breath control with daily activities, such as practicing mindful breathing during morning coffee or evening wind-down rituals.

3. Use Technology

Leverage apps like **Headspace** or **Calm** that offer guided breathing exercises and reminders to practice throughout the day.

4. Join a Community

Engage with local yoga or meditation groups to stay motivated and receive support from like-minded individuals.

5. Track Your Progress

Maintain a journal to note changes in your stress levels, emotional state, and overall well-being as you continue your breath mastery journey.

Achieving Mastery

Mastering your breath requires daily practice and mindfulness. It is a skill that, like any other, improves over time with consistent effort. As you practice these techniques, you will notice a gradual increase in your ability to manage stress, anxiety, and overwhelming emotions. You will also experience a deeper connection between your body and mind, as breath mastery facilitates emotional regulation and self-awareness.

As modern science catches up with ancient wisdom, it is clear that breath is more than just a physiological process. It is a tool for mental clarity, emotional stability, and trauma healing. The power to control your mental state lies quite literally in your breath. Through its mastery, you gain control over your emotions, your reactions, and ultimately, your life.

Victor O. Carl

Law 31

Write Your Story

"There is no greater agony than bearing an untold story inside you."— Maya Angelou

The Pen is Mightier When Used to Understand Oneself. Writing has long been hailed as one of the most powerful tools for self-reflection and emotional healing. Whether it's through journaling, storytelling, or simple note-taking, the act of putting thoughts to paper can serve as a profound method for processing trauma, understanding emotions, and ultimately, gaining control over one's mental state. This law emphasizes the importance of writing as a therapeutic tool—a way to externalize inner turmoil and transform chaotic thoughts into something tangible and understandable.

The Science Behind Writing as Therapy

Research in psychology and neuroscience supports the therapeutic benefits of writing. Studies have shown that expressive writing— where individuals write about their thoughts and feelings related to traumatic experiences—can lead to significant improvements in mental and physical health. Dr. James Pennebaker, a pioneer in this field, conducted studies that demonstrated how writing about trauma and emotional upheaval can enhance immune function, reduce stress, and lead to greater psychological well-being. His work revealed that those who write about their deepest thoughts and feelings for just 15-20 minutes a day, over the course of a few days, show significant health improvements months later.

One of Pennebaker's studies involved asking participants to write

167

about their most traumatic life experiences for four consecutive days. The results were remarkable: those who engaged in this writing exercise visited doctors less frequently, had better immune function, and experienced reduced levels of stress and anxiety compared to those who wrote about neutral topics. This study and others like it highlight how writing can serve as a release valve for pent-up emotions and unresolved trauma, helping individuals make sense of their experiences and regain control over their lives.

Writing as a Tool for Gaining Clarity

Writing allows individuals to distance themselves from their experiences, providing a new perspective on their thoughts and feelings. When you write, you're not just recounting events; you're engaging in a process of reflection and interpretation. This can help clarify emotions that might otherwise remain confusing or overwhelming. For example, when you write about a difficult experience, you may begin to see patterns in your behavior, identify triggers for certain emotions, or recognize connections between past and present challenges.

A study published in the journal *Psychological Science* found that people who wrote about their thoughts and feelings regarding a traumatic experience were able to better organize and structure their thoughts, which led to improved emotional clarity. This process of organizing thoughts on paper helps to reduce the mental load, making it easier to navigate complex emotions and reduce the intensity of trauma-related stress.

The Power of Narrative in Healing

Narrative therapy, a therapeutic approach developed by Michael White and David Epston, is based on the idea that we make sense of our lives through the stories we tell about ourselves. By rewriting these stories, we can change the way we perceive our experiences and, in turn, our lives. This therapeutic approach encourages individuals to externalize their problems—seeing them as separate from their identity—and then re-author their stories in a way that promotes healing and empowerment.

In a similar vein, keeping a journal or writing about personal experiences can help individuals create a coherent narrative of their lives. This narrative not only helps to make sense of past events but also empowers individuals to see themselves as active agents in their own stories. Instead of being defined by trauma, they can redefine their experiences, emphasizing their resilience, growth, and the lessons learned along the way.

Practical Steps to Writing Your Story

1. **Set Aside Time for Writing:** Make writing a regular part of your routine. Whether it's daily, weekly, or whenever you feel the need, setting aside dedicated time to write can help you make sense of your thoughts and emotions.
2. **Start with Free Writing:** Begin by writing without any specific structure or goal in mind. Let your thoughts flow freely onto the paper. This can help you access deeper emotions and uncover hidden feelings.
3. **Focus on Specific Experiences:** If you're dealing with a particular trauma or emotional issue, focus your writing on that experience. Describe what happened, how it made you feel, and what thoughts it triggered. Over time, you may begin to see patterns or insights emerge.
4. **Reflect on Your Writing:** After writing, take some time to read over what you've written. Reflect on any new insights or emotions that have come up. Consider how these insights might help you move forward or change your perspective.
5. **Reframe Negative Narratives:** If you notice that your writing is focused on negative aspects of your experiences, try to reframe the narrative. Focus on your strengths, the lessons you've learned, or the ways you've grown from the experience.

6. **Share Your Writing (If Comfortable):** Sometimes, sharing your writing with a trusted friend, therapist, or support group can provide additional insights and support. It can also help to verbalize your experiences and receive feedback from others.

Writing your story is more than just an exercise in putting words on paper; it's a powerful tool for self-discovery, healing, and transformation. By taking the time to write about your experiences, you can gain clarity on your emotions, process trauma, and begin to rewrite the narrative of your life in a way that empowers and heals. Whether you choose to keep a journal, write letters to yourself, or even craft stories or poems, the act of writing can be a key part of your journey toward mental and emotional well-being. Remember, the pen truly is mightier when used to understand oneself.

Law 32

Recognize Your Strength

"Our greatest glory is not in never falling, but in rising every time we fall." — Confucius

Your past victories are not just memories but are crucial markers of your resilience. In the aftermath of trauma, it's easy to feel defeated, but it's important to remember that surviving such experiences is itself a testament to your strength. Recognizing and honoring that resilience can pave the way to healing and empowerment.

Understanding Resilience in the Face of Trauma

Resilience, often defined as the ability to recover from adversity, is not something one is simply born with—it is built over time. Research on trauma survivors has shown that resilience is a complex interplay between personal factors and external support systems. For example, studies on individuals who have experienced traumatic events, such as natural disasters or personal violence, have found that those who actively engage in recovery efforts, such as helping others or participating in community rebuilding, have a much lower risk of long-term trauma effects compared to those who feel immobilized by their experiences.

A 2017 study published in the *Journal of Traumatic Stress* found that individuals who took part in community-driven recovery efforts after Hurricane Katrina exhibited higher levels of psychological resilience compared to those who did not participate. By engaging in meaningful action, these individuals were able to utilize their stress hormones, which are naturally secreted in response to trauma, for their intended purpose: to promote survival.

Stress hormones, such as cortisol and adrenaline, are often blamed for illness, but they are critical for survival when properly channeled. In response to extreme situations, they provide the body with the energy needed to react and cope. The issue arises when these hormones are not utilized, as seen in cases of immobilization or helplessness. When individuals feel trapped or unable to act, the stress hormones continue to circulate, leading to long-term physical and mental health issues, such as chronic anxiety or depression.

The Power of Action

Engaging in action is essential to harnessing the power of resilience. For those who feel immobilized, body-based therapies such as **somatic experiencing** and **sensorimotor psychotherapy** have been developed by experts like Peter Levine and Pat Ogden to help individuals reconnect with their body's innate ability to process trauma. These therapies focus on using physical sensations to guide recovery, enabling people to gradually expand their tolerance to distressing emotions and sensations.

Levine's concept of **pendulation**—the process of moving in and out of traumatic memories while focusing on physical sensations—allows individuals to gently confront their trauma without becoming overwhelmed. Over time, this practice builds resilience by increasing the individual's capacity to handle stress and reconnect with their body's natural fight-or-flight responses.

Rewriting the Narrative

Recognizing your strength begins by understanding that trauma does not define you. The brain, when exposed to trauma, may become stuck in a loop of fear or helplessness. However, modern neuroscience shows that the brain is incredibly adaptable and capable of rewriting old patterns. This ability, known as **neuroplasticity**, is what enables survivors of trauma to develop new coping mechanisms and emerge stronger.

Pierre Janet, a pioneering psychologist in the study of trauma, spoke about the "pleasure of completed action." This refers to the deep satisfaction individuals experience when they physically engage in completing the actions they were once immobilized from taking during a traumatic event. Through therapies like somatic experiencing, survivors are able to simulate the actions they were unable to complete, such as defending themselves or escaping danger. This not only resolves lingering trauma but also restores a sense of control and agency over their own lives.

In one powerful case study, a woman who had endured years of childhood abuse enrolled in a **model mugging** program. This program, originally developed in the 1970s, teaches individuals— especially women—how to fight back during a simulated attack. The experience helped her reclaim her sense of strength. Months later, when she was confronted by potential assailants, she confidently took a defensive stance and yelled, "Who wants to take me on first?" The attackers fled, recognizing her power.

This kind of confidence comes from understanding that strength is not about never being afraid or vulnerable; it's about how you handle those moments of vulnerability and rise beyond them.

How to Achieve This Law

1. **Acknowledge Your Past Victories**

Take time to reflect on the challenges you've overcome. Whether big or small, each obstacle you've faced contributes to your overall resilience. Journaling or creating a timeline of these moments can help you visualize your growth.

2. Engage in Active Recovery

Channel your stress into meaningful action. This could be anything from volunteering to helping others in distress, participating in physical activities, or even practicing mindfulness and yoga. Physical engagement helps the body process stress and prevents feelings of helplessness from taking hold.

3. Seek Somatic Healing

Explore therapies like somatic experiencing, which focus on reconnecting with your body. These methods help to release trapped emotions and complete the "incomplete" actions your body wanted to take during a traumatic event.

4. Embrace Neuroplasticity

Understand that the brain is not static. With the right tools, you can rewrite your responses to stress and trauma. Mindfulness meditation, cognitive behavioral therapy (CBT), and physical exercises all contribute to brain resilience.

Law 32 of Mental Power, **"Recognize Your Strength,"** reminds us that our past victories are evidence of the resilience that resides within us. Surviving trauma is not a sign of weakness, but a testament to the strength that lives within. By acknowledging that strength, taking action, and engaging in therapies that reconnect you with your body, you can move from a place of survival to thriving. Embrace your resilience, for it has carried you this far and will continue to be your greatest asset.

Law 33

Rebuild Trust Slowly

"The best way to find out if you can trust somebody is to trust them." - Ernest Hemingway

Trust is a fragile thing, but it can be mended; Trust is often shattered by trauma. Rebuilding it—both in yourself and in others—takes time, but it's essential for restoring healthy relationships.

Trust is like a delicate thread—once broken, it cannot simply be tied back together without visible knots and weaknesses. Trauma, betrayal, and deep emotional wounds often sever trust, leaving us wary, hurt, and isolated. However, despite the fragility of trust, it can be rebuilt—albeit slowly, methodically, and with care. Rebuilding trust is a crucial part of healing from trauma, essential for restoring healthy relationships, and most importantly, for rediscovering trust in oneself.

When trust is broken, the first reaction is often withdrawal—an attempt to protect oneself from further harm. This reaction is instinctive and can lead to feelings of isolation, fear, and anger. Studies show that trust is one of the most difficult things to regain once lost. Research from the American Psychological Association shows that trust issues stemming from trauma are deeply ingrained, and often tied to early experiences of betrayal or abandonment. In a study conducted by Harvard University, individuals who had experienced significant trauma were shown to have higher levels of distrust and anxiety when engaging with others, even years after the trauma occurred.

But why is trust so fragile? It's rooted in our most primal survival instincts. Trust allows us to feel safe, secure, and connected. When it's shattered, the very foundation of our relationships and our sense of self can feel threatened. Trauma can make the world appear dangerous, leading us to expect betrayal even from those who mean us no harm. A study published in THE JOURNAL OF TRAUMATIC STRESS found that people who had been through traumatic experiences often struggled with trusting their own judgment, as well as the intentions of others, further complicating their ability to form meaningful connections.

One of the essential steps in rebuilding trust is recognizing that it's a process, not a singular act. Trust, once broken, cannot be restored with grand gestures or promises. Instead, it's built piece by piece, over time. The body's response to trauma is a telling example of this. When we experience extreme stress or danger, our body secretes stress hormones like cortisol and adrenaline, meant to protect us in moments of crisis. However, when we are unable to act or escape—when we're immobilized or overwhelmed—these hormones can turn against us, creating patterns of hypervigilance and mistrust. Rebuilding trust requires re-regulating these systems and relearning how to feel safe again.

The Science Behind Trust and Trauma

Studies in the fields of psychology and neuroscience illustrate the intricate relationship between trauma and trust. Trauma can activate the body's stress response, flooding the brain with stress hormones like cortisol and adrenaline, which are meant to protect us in moments of danger. However, when these hormones are not properly utilized—such as in situations of helplessness or immobilization—they can lead to prolonged states of fear and distrust.

One study from the National Institute of Mental Health found that individuals with unresolved trauma often struggle with social interactions and trusting others, even when the threat has long passed. The brain's amygdala, responsible for processing fear, remains overactive, making it difficult for traumatized individuals to distinguish between real and perceived threats. As a result, the ability to trust—both in others and in oneself—is compromised.

Case Study: Rebuilding Trust After Trauma

Consider the example of a woman who had been in an abusive relationship. After years of enduring physical and emotional abuse, her ability to trust others—and herself—was shattered. Therapy became a lifeline, but progress was slow. Initially, she struggled to trust her therapist, doubting their intentions and fearing further harm. Over time, through consistent and safe interactions, she began to develop a sense of trust, not only in her therapist but also in her own ability to make decisions and set boundaries.

Gradually, she started to reconnect with friends and family, building trust one step at a time. Each positive experience reinforced the notion that trust could be rebuilt, though it required patience. She learned to identify red flags, communicate her needs clearly, and trust her gut instincts. Rebuilding trust in herself allowed her to navigate relationships with confidence, ultimately leading to healthier, more fulfilling connections.

Scientific Evidence Supporting Trust Recovery

A study published in NATURE HUMAN BEHAVIOUR highlighted the power of small, incremental trust-building exercises. In the study, participants were more likely to rebuild trust after a betrayal when the offender consistently engaged in small acts of kindness and reliability, compared to grand apologies or gestures. This research aligns with the principle that trust, once broken, is best repaired slowly through consistent, trustworthy actions over time.

Another powerful example comes from international peace efforts, where rebuilding trust between opposing groups has been critical to the process of reconciliation. The Northern Ireland peace process, for instance, demonstrated how long-standing distrust could be healed through consistent efforts of mutual cooperation and open dialogue, over the years. It highlights that trust isn't rebuilt overnight, but through patient, ongoing efforts.

In conclusion, Law 33 teaches us that trust is not a given—it is earned, fragile, and precious. Trauma may break it, but with time, patience, and consistent effort, trust can be rebuilt, both in others and in ourselves. Understanding that trust is rebuilt slowly helps us approach relationships with empathy, patience, and a deep sense of resilience. We learn to create a foundation where trust can flourish again, stronger and more resilient than before.

How to Rebuild Trust: A Step-by-Step Approach

1. **Acknowledge the Pain**: Recognizing that trust has been broken and accepting the emotions that come with it— anger, fear, and hurt—is the first step. Denial or avoidance only prolongs the healing process. Acknowledge the wound and understand that healing takes time.
2. **Start with Small Acts of Trust**: Begin by taking small steps. This might involve sharing a little more than you're

comfortable with, testing the waters, and observing how others respond. Don't rush into full trust all at once. Instead, offer it in small, manageable amounts, allowing others to demonstrate their reliability.

3. **Focus on Consistency**: Consistency is key to rebuilding trust. Trust is strengthened through repeated actions over time. A 2016 study in PERSONALITY AND SOCIAL PSYCHOLOGY BULLETIN revealed that consistent, reliable behavior was the strongest predictor of trust recovery in relationships. Show up, follow through on promises, and be reliable.

4. **Understand the Role of Boundaries**: Establishing clear boundaries is essential in protecting yourself while learning to trust again. Boundaries create a space where you feel safe, respected, and in control. When others honor your boundaries, trust begins to grow. Conversely, when boundaries are crossed, trust is further eroded.

5. **Communicate Openly**: Rebuilding trust requires honest communication. If trust has been broken, express how you feel in a non-confrontational way. This helps the other person understand the impact of their actions and shows your willingness to rebuild the relationship.

6. **Forgive, but Don't Forget**: Forgiveness is a vital part of the healing process, but it doesn't mean forgetting. Forgiveness allows you to release the burden of pain and anger, but it's also important to learn from the experience. Forgiveness is for your healing, not an excuse for repeated betrayals.

7. **Trust Yourself First**: Often, the most challenging part of rebuilding trust is learning to trust yourself again. Trauma can make you doubt your instincts and judgment, but reclaiming trust in yourself is crucial. This might involve trusting your ability to set boundaries, make decisions, or discern who is safe to trust.

In trauma recovery therapies like Somatic Experiencing, the concept of "renegotiation" is central to learning how to rebuild trust. This approach focuses on gradually re-engaging with the body's natural responses to stress. As one moves through the cycles of trauma and healing, individuals begin to trust their body's signals again, regaining a sense of safety and control. By re-experiencing physical sensations in a controlled environment, trauma survivors can learn that their body's natural responses are trustworthy, and they won't be overwhelmed by fear or immobilization. This process mirrors the slow, cautious rebuilding of trust in relationships—testing the waters, retreating when necessary, and gradually expanding one's capacity to trust over time.

Law 34

Eliminate the Toxic

"You don't have to let that toxic person rule your life. You can get rid of them. You can start right now." — Steve Maraboli

Toxicity, whether in relationships, environments, or habits, acts as a silent but pervasive force that hinders healing and growth. Just like physical toxins pollute the body, emotional and mental toxins disrupt our inner balance, preventing us from thriving. Toxic influences, much like environmental pollutants, cloud our ability to move forward and become our best selves. Removing them is not merely a suggestion—it is essential for your recovery and personal growth.

The Impact of Toxic Environments

Research in psychology and sociology has long demonstrated the powerful effects of our surroundings on our mental and emotional well-being. In a landmark 2006 study conducted by Dr. Sheldon Cohen at Carnegie Mellon University, the effects of chronic stress—often originating from toxic environments or relationships—were shown to weaken the immune system, making people more susceptible to illnesses. This study confirmed what many have long suspected: persistent stress from negative relationships and environments deteriorates both mental and physical health. The toxicity you allow in your life creates an environment where stress, anxiety, and trauma thrive.

This finding is further supported by a study published in the *Journal*

Victor O. Carl

181

of Social and Personal Relationships, which found that individuals in toxic relationships are more likely to suffer from depression, anxiety, and emotional distress. These relationships drain energy and stunt emotional growth, leaving individuals stuck in cycles of pain. Just as a plant needs fertile soil to grow, humans require positive and nurturing environments to thrive. Toxicity acts like poisoned soil, preventing growth.

How Trauma and Toxicity Are Linked

Trauma survivors often find themselves more vulnerable to toxic environments because trauma can distort self-worth and set the stage for toxic people or environments to take root. Dr. Peter Levine, a renowned trauma specialist, emphasizes in his work that unresolved trauma often creates a pattern where individuals are drawn to familiar but damaging situations. The trauma imprints on their psyche, making them more prone to tolerate toxicity. Toxicity and trauma are often intertwined, creating a cycle that is difficult to break unless addressed consciously and actively.

One fascinating element of trauma healing is found in Dr. Levine's *Somatic Experiencing* method. He notes that individuals who have unresolved trauma frequently feel "frozen," unable to escape toxic cycles. However, once they learn to recognize and honor their body's natural responses to danger, they can reclaim their power and eliminate toxic influences from their lives. This understanding is key to breaking free from toxic patterns that perpetuate suffering.

Breaking the Cycle: Steps to Eliminate Toxicity

1. **Identify the Source of Toxicity**
   To begin the process of eliminating toxicity, it's crucial to identify the toxic influences in your life. Toxicity can come from different sources: relationships that drain you emotionally, environments that suffocate your creativity, or habits that contribute to negative mental states. The

first step is acknowledging where the poison lies. Without identifying it, there can be no elimination.

Research in cognitive behavioral therapy (CBT) highlights that awareness is the first step toward change. Once you become aware of how toxic relationships or environments affect you, you can begin to take steps to eliminate them.

2. **Set Boundaries and Create Distance**
   Boundaries are the most effective defense against toxicity. Whether in personal relationships or professional environments, learning to say "no" and protect your emotional energy is key to removing the poison. A 2017 study published in *Personality and Social Psychology Bulletin* found that individuals who maintain strong emotional boundaries report higher levels of self-esteem and life satisfaction.

   Boundaries are essential to reclaiming your emotional space and preventing toxic influences from reentering your life. Start small, like limiting exposure to negative conversations or reducing time spent with toxic individuals. Gradually, as you feel stronger, you can create a more substantial distance.

3. **Replace the Toxic with the Positive**
   Once you begin to eliminate the toxic influences, you must fill that space with positive, uplifting elements. Surround yourself with people who uplift and support you, create a nurturing home environment, and adopt habits that contribute to your emotional and physical well-being. According to the *Harvard Study of Adult Development*, which followed participants for over 80 years, one of the key predictors of happiness and longevity was the presence of healthy relationships.

   Positive influences nourish your mental health, providing the fertile ground for healing. It's not enough to just remove the poison—you must actively cultivate what is healthy and beneficial to replace it.

Practical Case Studies: The Power of Elimination

- ### Case Study 1: Bob Barklay's Heroism

In a crisis where Bob and other children were trapped in an underground vault, Bob's focused energy helped minimize the traumatic effects of the event. By remaining engaged in the task of freeing himself and others, Bob was able to channel his nervous energy in a productive way, reducing the long-term effects of trauma. This exemplifies the importance of action and focus in trauma recovery. Like Bob, eliminating toxic influences from our lives requires intentional effort and sustained focus on removing what holds us back.

- ### Case Study 2: Nancy's Liberation

After a traumatic tonsillectomy experience, Nancy reawakened her capacity for healing by simulating the escape movements she had suppressed during her trauma. This movement freed her from the lingering effects of the trauma, showing that active engagement in healing processes— whether through physical movement, therapy, or boundary- setting—releases trapped energy and restores balance. Nancy's story demonstrates that eliminating toxic influences, whether emotional or physical, requires proactive action to break free.

Achieving Law 34: Eliminate the Toxic

1. **Recognize the Toxic Influences**: The first step to eliminating the toxic is becoming aware of what or who is causing the negativity. Reflect on your relationships, environment, and habits. Identify what drains your energy, triggers stress, or holds you back.

2. **Set Boundaries**: Setting boundaries is essential to protect yourself from further harm. Limit your interactions with toxic people, avoid environments that breed negativity, and prioritize your well-being over others' expectations.
3. **Seek Support**: Healing is often a collaborative process. Surround yourself with positive, supportive people who encourage your growth. This might include friends, family, therapists, or support groups. Positive reinforcement accelerates healing.
4. **Replace Toxicity with Positivity**: As you remove the toxic influences, replace them with activities, people, and habits that nurture you. Engage in practices like mindfulness, physical activity, and creativity, which foster positive energy and emotional well-being.
5. **Practice Patience and Persistence**: Removing toxic influences is not always easy and often takes time. Be patient with yourself and the process. Every small step you take is progress toward a healthier, more fulfilling life.

Law 34 teaches us that just as our bodies cannot heal in toxic environments, our minds and spirits also require a healthy space to recover. Eliminating the toxic is not an act of selfishness but one of self-preservation and growth. By identifying the toxins in our lives and taking action to remove them, we create space for healing, self-discovery, and personal transformation. The journey may be gradual, but each step leads to a life free from the poison that once held you back.

Law 35

Learn the Science

"Until you make the unconscious conscious, it will direct your life and you will call it fate."- Carl Jung

Understanding trauma unlocks the door to recovery. Grasping the physiological and psychological effects of trauma demystifies your experiences and empowers your recovery.

Trauma is an invisible force that influences our lives in ways that many fail to comprehend. What we don't know about it can, and often does, hurt us. Trauma manifests in various forms, from overwhelming anxiety and emotional numbness to physical symptoms that leave many searching for answers. By not understanding trauma, we risk mistaking its effects for personal failings, weaknesses, or untreatable conditions.

The research underscores this. Studies have shown that trauma victims often experience chronic stress responses that affect both their mental and physical health. The *Adverse Childhood Experiences (ACE) Study*, one of the largest investigations of childhood trauma, revealed that individuals with high ACE scores were significantly more likely to suffer from chronic diseases, depression, and even premature death. Understanding trauma from a scientific perspective allows us to grasp the biological and psychological mechanisms at play and demystify our seemingly irrational reactions.

The Physiology of Trauma

Trauma rewires the brain, primarily impacting the limbic system—the seat of emotion. When faced with trauma, the brain's stress circuits activate the "fight, flight, or freeze" responses, leaving the body in a constant state of hyperarousal. The amygdala, which regulates fear, becomes hyperactive, while the prefrontal cortex—the rational part of the brain—diminishes in influence, making it hard for trauma survivors to process emotions logically.

Understanding this neurological process is crucial. Brain imaging studies, such as those by *Dr. Bessel van der Kolk*, have demonstrated how trauma alters the brain's structure. These changes explain why trauma survivors may react disproportionately to small triggers or feel disconnected from their bodies. When you understand that these reactions are not personal failures but neurological responses, the shame and confusion often accompanying trauma can begin to dissipate.

The Psychological Impact

Psychologically, trauma can distort memory and create fragmented, confusing experiences that haunt the mind. The *DSM-5* (Diagnostic and Statistical Manual of Mental Disorders) acknowledges that trauma can lead to disorders like PTSD, where individuals constantly relive traumatic events through flashbacks, nightmares, or intrusive thoughts. Yet, trauma's impact is not limited to the mind; it often manifests physically. Studies by *Harvard University* have found that trauma survivors are more likely to develop autoimmune diseases, chronic pain, and even heart problems due to prolonged exposure to stress hormones like cortisol.

How do we use this knowledge to heal?

The Path to Recovery

1. **Education as Empowerment:**The first step in healing from trauma is understanding it. This involves educating

yourself about the physiological and psychological effects of trauma. Books like *The Body Keeps the Score* by Dr. Bessel van der Kolk explain how trauma lodges itself in both the body and the mind, offering a scientific framework for recovery. When you understand that trauma manifests through a series of automatic, bodily responses, you can start shifting from victimhood to empowerment.

2. **A Mind-Body Approach:**Trauma is not solely a mental phenomenon; it deeply affects the body. Practices like yoga, mindfulness, and somatic therapy work to reconnect the body and mind. Research published in the *Journal of Traumatic Stress* shows that yoga and mindfulness can significantly reduce PTSD symptoms by restoring the brain's ability to regulate emotions. These techniques help bring awareness to the body, allowing individuals to process trauma without being overwhelmed.

3. **Shamanic and Communal Healing:**Throughout history, shamanic cultures have understood trauma as a community issue. They believed that trauma fragments the soul and that healing requires communal support to restore balance. While modern Western practices often overlook this communal aspect, research shows that support networks are one of the strongest predictors of recovery. Survivors who have a close network of family, friends, or group therapy tend to heal more quickly. Embracing this knowledge, trauma survivors should actively seek communities that offer understanding and safety.

4. **Neurofeedback and Cognitive Behavioral Therapy (CBT):**Cutting-edge treatments like neurofeedback and CBT help to restore balance in the brain. *Neurofeedback* is a technology that trains the brain to self-regulate, significantly reducing trauma symptoms by reestablishing proper neural connections. CBT, on the other hand, provides survivors with tools to reframe their thoughts and break free from destructive patterns.

Applying Law 35: Learn the Science

By learning the science behind trauma, we begin to reclaim our lives. We move from confusion and helplessness to a place of empowerment. This understanding not only removes the shame often associated with trauma but also gives survivors a clear roadmap to recovery.

Practical Steps to Achieve This Law

- **Education:** Dive deep into trauma literature to understand the biological and psychological mechanisms. Knowledge is the first step to healing.
- **Mind-Body Practices:** Incorporate yoga, mindfulness, and breathwork into your daily routine to soothe the nervous system and reconnect with your body.
- **Seek Professional Help:** Utilize trauma-informed therapies like EMDR (Eye Movement Desensitization and Reprocessing) and CBT to address deep-rooted trauma in a safe and structured way.
- **Build a Support Network:** Surround yourself with a community that provides empathy, safety, and support. Healing in isolation is far more difficult than healing with communal support.

Learning the science behind trauma is the key to unlocking the door to recovery. When we understand how trauma affects the brain and body, we begin to demystify its grip on our lives. We stop viewing our symptoms as personal failings and instead see them as responses to past events that can be understood, addressed, and healed.

Law 36

Give Back to Heal

"I don't know what your destiny will be, but one thing I know: the only ones among you who will be really happy are those who have sought and found how to serve." - Albert Schweitzer

When we are trapped in the whirlwind of our own pain, it can feel as though nothing will ever alleviate the weight we carry. However, countless studies and real-world examples show that one of the most profound ways to heal yourself is through helping others. This law taps into a timeless principle that by serving others, we rediscover purpose, reawaken dormant strengths, and initiate a process of healing within ourselves. The road to personal recovery is often paved with the good we do for others.

Several studies in the field of psychology suggest that when we help others, we activate areas of our brain associated with pleasure and reward. This phenomenon, sometimes referred to as the **"helper's high,"** occurs when our brains release dopamine and oxytocin—the feel-good hormones—as a reward for doing good. Not only do these hormones improve mood, but they also lower stress and anxiety levels, thus promoting physical and emotional healing.

A study published by *United Health Group* in 2017 found that 76% of people who volunteered in some capacity felt healthier overall, and 94% of volunteers reported an improved mood and higher self-esteem after engaging in service activities. This psychological shift is more than just a brief uplift; it can become a long-term strategy for managing one's emotional well-being.

The Science of Purpose

Understanding how giving back creates a sense of purpose is rooted in the science of human motivation. Viktor Frankl, the famous psychologist and Holocaust survivor, captured this idea in his seminal work, *Man's Search for Meaning,* where he explained that purpose is a cornerstone of human survival, even in the most difficult of circumstances. Finding a cause outside ourselves connects us to a larger framework of meaning. It realigns our suffering within the broader human experience and provides a way to process and transcend it.

Studies conducted by the *National Institute on Aging* found that individuals who report having a strong sense of purpose live longer, healthier lives. These individuals also showed lower levels of inflammatory markers, which are linked to chronic diseases such as heart disease and cancer. Having a purpose—especially one that involves helping others—stimulates the body's natural resilience, making both emotional and physical recovery more achievable.

Real-World Examples

One of the most illustrative cases of the healing power of giving back comes from the life of **Oprah Winfrey**. Growing up in extreme poverty and surviving multiple traumas, including sexual abuse, Winfrey rose to become one of the most influential media figures in the world. However, she attributes much of her healing and sense of personal fulfillment to her philanthropic work, particularly with young girls in South Africa through her leadership academy. By lifting others up, she created a sense of fulfillment and healing that transcended her personal suffering.

Similarly, **James Doty**, a neurosurgeon and author of *Into the Magic Shop*, grew up in an environment filled with abuse, poverty, and uncertainty. Doty found healing and meaning in his work serving others, not only through his profession but also through philanthropy, creating initiatives to support children from underserved communities. His ability to focus outward helped him rebuild his sense of identity and purpose.

In the world of veterans, **Team Rubicon** serves as a powerful example. Founded by former Marines and veterans, Team Rubicon uses the skills learned in combat to deploy aid in disaster zones worldwide. Many of the veterans involved in this organization report that helping others gave them a renewed sense of purpose and aided in their transition back into civilian life. Research conducted by *Syracuse University's Institute for Veterans and Military Families* found that veterans who engaged in volunteer work were 27% less likely to experience depression and anxiety than their counterparts who didn't.

The Ripple Effect of Giving Back

The effect of helping others extends far beyond the individual. When you give back, you create a ripple effect that can transform entire communities. The *Harvard Business School* conducted a study that found people who give their time or resources to others tend to inspire others around them to do the same, multiplying the benefits of goodwill.

When you serve others, you are not only supporting their healing journey but also creating a cycle of reciprocity. Communities that engage in mutual support show higher rates of recovery, lower levels of mental illness, and a greater overall sense of well-being.

How to Achieve Law 36: Practical Steps

1. **Start Small, Stay Consistent:** You don't need to change the world overnight. Start by offering your time and skills to someone in need within your local community. Volunteering at a food bank, mentoring a youth, or even

spending time with isolated seniors can have a tremendous impact on both you and those you help.

2. **Leverage Your Strengths:** Think about what you're naturally good at or passionate about. If you're an artist, volunteer to teach art classes at a local community center. If you're an engineer, consider mentoring students or offering workshops. When you align your service with your skills, the act of giving becomes sustainable and fulfilling.

3. **Join a Group or Organization:** Find organizations that align with causes close to your heart. Whether it's environmental activism, mental health advocacy, or helping refugees, aligning yourself with a collective effort amplifies the impact of your contribution.

4. **Practice Empathy:** It's essential to give not just material help, but emotional support. Listening, offering words of encouragement, and showing understanding can be some of the most powerful gifts you can give someone in need.

5. **Reflect on Your Growth:** Take time to reflect on how giving back has influenced your own healing. Journaling, meditating, or speaking with a therapist can help you recognize the ways in which your service has transformed you, reinforcing the positive feedback loop of healing.

Law 36 emphasizes that healing is often found in service to others. Whether through small acts of kindness or larger commitments to philanthropy, helping others enables us to step outside of ourselves, find purpose, and initiate our healing journey. It is a profound way to not only give to others but also to nurture the parts of ourselves that need restoration.

In giving back, you heal. The science, statistics, and countless examples make it clear: service is not just a noble act; it is a path to your salvation.

Law 37

Turn Setbacks into Lessons

"The best way to find yourself is to lose yourself in the service of others."— Mahatma Gandhi

In serving others, you find your own salvation; helping those struggling can provide a sense of purpose and fulfillment, aiding in your healing journey.

Trauma is an isolating experience, often trapping individuals in cycles of pain, confusion, and emotional paralysis. But one of the most powerful pathways out of this isolation is through the act of service to others. Law 37, "Give Back to Heal," emphasizes that helping those in need can be the catalyst for personal recovery. This law underscores the transformative potential of extending a hand to others while simultaneously healing your own soul. Research supports the idea that giving back, especially through community and social engagement, provides not only emotional benefits but also physiological and mental health improvements.

Studies have shown that acts of altruism and service to others can significantly improve mental health. A comprehensive review by *Dr. Stephen Post* at Stony Brook University found that engaging in meaningful service reduces stress and increases overall life satisfaction. Helping others boosts the release of oxytocin, a hormone linked to feelings of warmth and connection, while simultaneously decreasing cortisol, the stress hormone. Furthermore, research published in *The Journal of Happiness Studies* revealed that those who regularly engaged in volunteer work reported lower rates of depression and higher rates of self-worth and fulfillment. These benefits come not from ignoring personal trauma but by transcending it—finding a higher purpose in aiding others.

Take the story of John Lewis, the U.S. civil rights leader who faced severe trauma during his fight for racial equality, including the notorious "Bloody Sunday" attack in Selma. Rather than retreating into his suffering, Lewis channeled his pain into helping others and fighting for justice. His deep commitment to improving the lives of marginalized people became his path to healing, giving his life profound meaning. His public service allowed him to transform personal trauma into societal change, illustrating how purpose-driven work can alleviate emotional scars.

The Physiological Impact of Service

Neuroscience also shows that engaging in altruistic behavior rewires the brain to support positive mental states. Acts of kindness, charity, or mentorship activate the brain's reward system, specifically, the mesolimbic pathway, which is associated with feelings of pleasure and fulfillment. This explains why many trauma survivors who engage in helping others often describe their experiences as deeply meaningful and healing.

When trauma is left unresolved, it can remain stuck in the body, as Peter Levine's work on somatic healing has demonstrated. This unprocessed trauma causes chronic stress responses—tight muscles, rapid heartbeat, or shallow breathing—similar to being in a state of constant fight or flight. Serving others can help disrupt these patterns, shifting the focus from internal suffering to external compassion. This shift engages the parasympathetic nervous system, responsible for promoting calmness and reducing the physiological burden of stress.

Healing Through Giving

There are countless examples of individuals who have found healing by helping others. In the aftermath of the 2010 Haiti earthquake, trauma psychologist *Danielle Rousseau* noted a significant increase in psychological resilience among those who provided relief aid. Individuals who initially felt helpless in their own pain found solace and healing by helping earthquake survivors rebuild their lives. The shared experience of suffering—and mutual acts of giving—created a space where trauma could be processed in a community rather than in isolation.

Similarly, combat veterans often find meaning in service to fellow veterans. Organizations like *Team Rubicon*, which mobilizes veterans to respond to disasters, have witnessed firsthand how soldiers dealing with PTSD experience improved mental health outcomes by engaging in purposeful action. This type of giving allows veterans to rediscover a sense of agency, camaraderie, and contribution—elements often stripped away by trauma.

Achieving Law 37: How to Give Back and Heal

1. **Start Small and Local**
    Healing through service doesn't require monumental efforts. Begin by identifying small acts of kindness or opportunities to volunteer in your community. Whether it's assisting in a local shelter or mentoring a young person, even minor acts of service can activate your brain's reward system and foster feelings of connection and purpose.

2. **Focus on Shared Experiences**
If you've experienced trauma, consider helping those with similar struggles. Peer support networks are powerful healing tools. Programs like *Alcoholics Anonymous* and *Veterans Peer Support Groups* demonstrate how shared experiences can turn personal pain into a source of strength for others. By using your story to uplift others, you often find your own sense of peace and recovery.

3. **Integrate Service into Routine**
Consistency is key. Research shows that those who regularly engage in helping others reap more long-term psychological and physiological benefits. Make service a regular part of your life, whether it's a weekly commitment or something more frequent.

4. **Mentorship and Purposeful Work**
Giving back can be as simple as offering mentorship. Studies from *The Harvard T.H. Chan School of Public Health* have shown that older adults who mentor younger individuals feel a renewed sense of purpose and report lower levels of anxiety and depression. This applies to people at any stage of life; sharing knowledge or skills with someone in need strengthens both the mentor and mentee.

5. **Engage with Communities of Support**
Healing is often a communal process. Trauma isolates, but service connects. Whether through organized programs, faith-based organizations, or informal communities, engaging with a collective that is dedicated to service amplifies the healing effect.

Victor Frankl, the renowned Holocaust survivor and psychiatrist, famously stated: **"Those who have a 'why' to live can bear with almost any 'how.'"** His profound insight illuminates the heart of

Law 37: Giving back not only fosters healing in others, but it also gives you a reason to move beyond the pain of trauma. It reintroduces a sense of purpose and reminds you that you have something invaluable to offer the world.

By embracing this law, you embark on a journey of mutual healing—one where both you and those you help are transformed.

In serving others, you find not just solace but a pathway to reclaiming your own strength, purpose, and peace.

Law 38

Stay Open to New Beginnings

"Life is a series of natural and spontaneous changes. Don't resist them; that only creates sorrow. Let reality be reality. Let things flow naturally forward in whatever way they like."—
Lao Tzu

In life, we often resist change and retreat into what's familiar, especially after experiencing trauma. The comfort of the known is our mental fortress, protecting us from the unknown, which can feel like a vast ocean of uncertainty. Yet, if we stay closed off, we miss out on the many possibilities and growth opportunities that lie ahead.

When we talk about freedom, we often mean the freedom to choose—to live life on our terms. But true freedom is about more than just external circumstances; it is about the liberation of the human spirit. And for many of us, that spirit is often shackled by the past. Traumatic experiences, disappointments, or failures can create invisible walls around our hearts and minds, making us hesitant to embrace new beginnings.

We tend to blame the world for our lack of freedom. We point fingers at governments, circumstances, religion, or even fate. But the reality is, the greatest enemy to our freedom often resides within us. It is our own unwillingness to break old patterns, to step outside of the familiar, that holds us captive.

Research in psychology has shown that traumatic events can reshape our brains in ways that make us fearful of the unknown. A 2017 study published in *The Journal of Neuroscience* found that trauma alters the brain's fear circuitry, causing us to overestimate potential threats in new environments . This makes us cling to the old, even when it no longer serves us, because the mind has been programmed to equate familiarity with safety.

So how do we break free? How do we stay open to new beginnings despite the weight of our past?

The Key to Transformation: Awareness

The first step in embracing new beginnings is becoming aware that you're stuck in the past. Without awareness, there is no change. Imagine you're walking through a fog, unable to see clearly. In this fog, your decisions are based on outdated beliefs and fears. But once you recognize that your thinking is clouded, you can begin to clear the fog and open yourself up to fresh opportunities.

Becoming aware of your limiting beliefs—those agreements you made with yourself in response to past traumas—is essential. These are the silent contracts we sign, usually as children, without realizing it. For example, you might have agreed long ago that "I'm not good enough," or "I'll never succeed." These agreements form the foundation of your personal belief system and control your life, keeping you tethered to old ways of thinking and behaving.

The Transformation of Trauma into Growth

Let's take the example of Viktor Frankl, the Austrian psychiatrist and Holocaust survivor. In his seminal work *Man's Search for Meaning*, Frankl details how even in the face of unimaginable suffering, he was able to find purpose and meaning. Frankl's experience highlights that new beginnings can arise even in the darkest moments. It wasn't the physical circumstances of the concentration camp that determined his inner freedom; it was his mindset. He embraced the possibility that even this terrible trauma could offer new meaning .

Modern studies in *post-traumatic growth* echo Frankl's philosophy. According to research by psychologist Richard Tedeschi, people who undergo traumatic experiences often report a deeper appreciation of life, improved relationships, and an openness to new possibilities . They grow not *despite* their trauma, but *because of* it.

In order to stay open to new beginnings, you must first break the old agreements that keep you trapped in outdated beliefs. These are the agreements that tell you, "You're not good enough," "You'll fail," or "You can't trust people." These agreements were formed in response to past traumas and experiences, but they no longer serve you.

One way to start breaking these agreements is to question them. Ask yourself: Is this belief really true? Can I find evidence that contradicts it? By doing this, you create space for new beliefs to form, and this is where new beginnings take root.

Another powerful way to break old agreements is through self-forgiveness. Forgiving yourself for past mistakes or for letting others hurt you is like removing heavy chains from your spirit. Once those chains are lifted, you become free to explore new opportunities without the burden of guilt or shame.

The Power of Repetition and Growth

Change doesn't happen overnight. Old patterns are deeply ingrained, and breaking them requires continuous effort. Repetition is the key to mastery. Every time you choose a new path, you strengthen the neural pathways in your brain associated with growth and resilience. Neuroscientific studies show that the brain is highly plastic, meaning it can reorganize itself based on new experiences and behaviors .

By repeatedly exposing yourself to new experiences, no matter how small, you begin to rewire your brain for growth rather than survival. This doesn't mean you'll never feel fear or doubt again, but it does mean that you'll become more comfortable with uncertainty and open to the possibilities it brings.

Embracing the Unknown: Lessons from Nature

The natural world is full of examples of transformation and new beginnings. Think of a caterpillar, confined to the earth, destined only to crawl. It enters a dark cocoon, a place of transformation. Inside, it dissolves into a kind of biological soup, a process that seems like an ending. But in truth, it is the beginning of something far greater—the birth of a butterfly.

Just like the butterfly, you may find yourself in dark, uncertain places, but these moments of transformation are necessary. The cocoon of your old beliefs must dissolve so that you can spread your wings and soar into new beginnings.

How to Stay Open to New Beginnings

1. **Practice Mindfulness:** Becoming aware of your thoughts and emotions as they arise will help you identify old patterns and beliefs that no longer serve you. Meditation or journaling can be powerful tools to cultivate this awareness.
2. **Challenge Limiting Beliefs:** Regularly question the validity of your self-imposed limitations. Look for evidence that contradicts them and explore new perspectives.
3. **Embrace Uncertainty:** Learn to view uncertainty not as a threat but as an opportunity for growth. Every time you step into the unknown, you build your resilience and mental power.
4. **Repetition and Growth:** Keep practicing new behaviors and thinking patterns until they become second nature. Remember, change is a process, not a one-time event.

New beginnings are not the absence of struggle, but the ability to find growth and joy in the midst of it. Staying open to them requires breaking free from the chains of old agreements and embracing the unknown. When you choose to do this, the future becomes not something to fear, but a vast horizon of possibility.

And as the old saying goes: "What lies behind us and what lies before us are tiny matters compared to what lies within us.

Law 39

Build Resilience from Adversity

"The oak fought the wind and was broken, the willow bent when it must and survived."
— Robert Jordan

The strongest steel is forged in the hottest fire; Adversity builds resilience. Each challenge you overcome makes you stronger, preparing you for whatever lies ahead.

Adversity is often seen as something to avoid, a burden, or an obstacle. However, when we shift our perspective, we can view adversity as one of life's greatest teachers—a crucible that strengthens us, shapes us, and ultimately helps us build resilience. This resilience is the mental, emotional, and psychological strength that enables us to face challenges, adapt to difficult situations, and keep moving forward.

The ancient proverb, "The strongest steel is forged in the hottest fire," captures the essence of this idea. Resilience is not something we are born with but rather something developed through adversity. The fires of hardship have the potential to either break us or transform us, but the difference lies in how we approach and learn from these experiences.

The Science of Resilience: Understanding its Origins

Resilience, like any skill, can be nurtured and developed. Extensive studies in the fields of psychology and neuroscience have demonstrated that the human brain is malleable and can be conditioned to respond to adversity with strength rather than retreat. One groundbreaking study is the **Minnesota Longitudinal Study of Risk and Adaptation**, which tracked 180 children over 30 years to understand how early experiences with adversity affected their development.

The researchers found that the most significant factor in building resilience was not intelligence, temperament, or even economic status, but the quality of early caregiving. Children who had consistent, nurturing caregivers were more likely to become resilient adults, even when faced with significant adversity. The study concluded that resilience is born from relationships that foster emotional regulation, stability, and a sense of security.

Resilience in Action: The study also highlighted how children who faced neglect or inconsistent caregiving often developed anxiety, hyperactivity, and difficulty managing stress. In contrast, those who received emotional support and were encouraged to develop autonomy became better at regulating their emotions and coping with challenges.

Adversity as a Catalyst for Growth

A modern understanding of resilience goes beyond merely "bouncing back" from hardship; it involves growing stronger from it. Psychologist **Ann Masten** describes resilience as "ordinary magic"—the ability to adapt, learn, and grow despite challenges.

In a world filled with unpredictability, from global pandemics to economic crises, cultivating resilience is more crucial than ever. People who experience and overcome adversity often develop a heightened sense of self-efficacy and purpose. For instance, research on survivors of trauma has consistently shown that many emerge with a greater sense of purpose, often finding new meaning in life and developing an increased capacity for empathy and service to others.

Overcoming Adversity in Real Life

One notable example is **Viktor Frankl**, an Austrian neurologist and Holocaust survivor, who authored the renowned book *Man's Search for Meaning*. In it, Frankl describes how his experience in concentration camps taught him that, although suffering is inevitable, we have the power to choose how we respond to it. His philosophy of finding meaning through adversity became a cornerstone of modern psychological thought, showing that even in the most horrific circumstances, humans can grow stronger and more resilient.

Another powerful story of resilience comes from **Malala Yousafzai**, the Pakistani activist who was shot by the Taliban for advocating for girls' education. Despite nearly losing her life, Malala used the experience to fuel her activism, becoming a global symbol of resilience and courage. Her ability to transform a personal tragedy into a powerful movement demonstrates that adversity, while painful, can be a catalyst for growth and empowerment.

How to Build Resilience: Practical Steps

Building resilience is a process that involves cultivating habits, mindsets, and practices that fortify your mental strength. Here are several strategies, grounded in research, that can help you develop resilience:

1. **Develop Emotional Awareness and Regulation:** The ability to recognize and regulate your emotions is fundamental to resilience. Studies show that people who can identify their emotions and understand their triggers are better equipped to cope with adversity. Practicing mindfulness, meditation, or journaling can increase self-awareness and emotional regulation.

2. **Embrace a Growth Mindset**: The concept of the *growth mindset*, developed by psychologist **Carol Dweck**, emphasizes that abilities and intelligence can be developed with effort. Individuals who adopt this mindset view challenges as opportunities to grow rather than as threats. By seeing failure as a learning experience rather than a definitive end, you build the mental flexibility needed to handle setbacks.
3. **Build Strong Relationships**: As the Minnesota study demonstrated, relationships are key to resilience. Surrounding yourself with a supportive network of family, friends, and mentors creates a buffer against life's stressors. Seek out those who uplift you and be willing to ask for help when needed.
4. **Set Small, Achievable Goals**: Resilience is built through perseverance. Setting small, achievable goals helps you build momentum, which can foster confidence. Each small victory reinforces the idea that you can overcome obstacles, making future challenges less intimidating.
5. **Cultivate OptimismMartin Seligman**, the father of positive psychology, found that optimism plays a key role in resilience. Optimistic individuals are more likely to view setbacks as temporary and surmountable, whereas pessimistic individuals tend to see difficulties as permanent and insurmountable. By practicing gratitude and reframing negative experiences, you can train your mind to focus on the positives, even in difficult times.
6. **Practice Self-Compassion**: Resilience also involves being kind to yourself when you fail or encounter setbacks. **Kristin Neff's** research on self-compassion shows that individuals who practice self-compassion are less likely to be overwhelmed by failure and more likely to bounce back from adversity. Self-compassion allows you to view your challenges with greater perspective and patience.
7. **Embrace Physical Activity**: Engaging in regular physical exercise has been shown to reduce stress, increase mental clarity, and improve mood. Exercise boosts the production of neurotransmitters like endorphins and serotonin, which

are associated with improved emotional well-being, resilience, and overall mental health.

Resilience, like the strongest steel, is forged through hardship. Whether it's in facing personal challenges or societal difficulties, adversity is not just something to survive; it's something that can transform us into stronger, more capable individuals. By building emotional awareness, developing supportive relationships, setting achievable goals, and maintaining a growth mindset, we can turn life's challenges into opportunities for growth.

The path to resilience is not a straight line, but with each step, you are shaping yourself into someone who can not only withstand life's toughest moments but also thrive in their aftermath. In the words of **Helen Keller**, who triumphed over seemingly insurmountable   adversity:
"Although the world is full of suffering, it is also full of the overcoming of it."

Law 40

Live in the Now

"Do not dwell in the past, do not dream of the future, concentrate the mind on the present moment." — *Buddha*

The present moment is the only reality you truly control; The present moment is where healing occurs. Focus on the here and now to reduce anxiety and connect with your inner peace. Living in the present often referred to as *mindfulness*, is a concept deeply rooted in both ancient wisdom and modern psychology. It's the conscious decision to focus your attention on the now—free from past regrets or future anxieties. When you live in the now, you engage with life as it unfolds, leading to deeper connections with your own emotions, increased mental clarity, and improved physical well-being.

A growing body of research has shown that mindfulness can significantly improve mental health. A study conducted by Harvard researchers using fMRI scans revealed that mindfulness training increases the density of gray matter in the hippocampus, which is involved in learning and memory, and in other brain structures associated with self-awareness and emotional regulation. People who live in the present show lower activity in the amygdala, the brain's alarm system for stress and anxiety, leading to a reduction in the levels of cortisol and adrenaline—hormones linked to stress.

Additionally, studies from the National Institutes of Health found that those who practice mindfulness had reduced symptoms of anxiety, depression, and chronic pain. This occurs because mindfulness rewires the brain to better handle stress. As psychiatrist Judson Brewer describes, mindfulness is like *hacking* the brain's habitual stress responses by breaking the cycle of worry and anxiety, thereby redirecting the mind back to the present moment.

The Cost of Not Living in the Now

When individuals fail to live in the present, they often find themselves either trapped in the past, weighed down by regret and guilt, or lost in the future, consumed by anxiety and uncertainty. This "time-traveling mind" affects not only mental health but also physical well-being. Chronic stress resulting from constantly living outside of the present has been linked to high blood pressure, heart disease, and digestive problems. Living disconnected from the moment can also erode relationships, as it prevents people from fully engaging with others.

Consider the example of *Steve Jobs*, who was famously an advocate for mindfulness. Jobs incorporated Zen mindfulness practices into his life, which he credited for shaping his extraordinary creativity and resilience. His mindfulness practice helped him focus on the present, leading to some of the most transformative innovations in history, like the iPhone and iPad. It wasn't just about creating technology; it was about living with awareness and focus in each moment.

Historical Example: Marcus Aurelius

A less modern, yet equally compelling example, is *Marcus Aurelius*, the Roman Emperor, and Stoic philosopher. In his *Meditations*, Aurelius frequently reflected on the importance of living in the present. Despite facing immense challenges, including wars and plagues, he emphasized that life exists only in the moment and that by mastering one's own mind, one could achieve peace and clarity. His writings remain a guide for leaders and thinkers on how to live effectively in the present while managing overwhelming responsibilities.

Aurelius wrote: *"Confine yourself to the present."* His philosophy was built around accepting what you can't control and focusing your energy on what you can, which is your own mind and actions in the current moment. This is the essence of Law 40—learning to live within the space that you truly influence, the *now*.

How to Achieve This Law

1. **Practice Mindfulness Meditation**: One of the most effective methods for anchoring yourself in the present moment is mindfulness meditation. Start with just 10-15 minutes a day, focusing on your breath and the sensations in your body. Every time your mind wanders, gently guide it back to your breath. Over time, this practice strengthens your ability to stay present.
2. **Develop Sensory Awareness**: Engage your senses deliberately. Whether it's savoring a meal, listening to music, or feeling the breeze on your skin, draw your attention to the sensations around you. This keeps you connected to the here and now.
3. **Embrace Gratitude**: Gratitude naturally draws your attention to the present. By appreciating what you have at this moment, you shift your focus away from what you lack or fear. Keeping a gratitude journal can reinforce this habit, promoting a mindset that values the present.
4. **Let Go of Perfectionism**: Many people are future-oriented because they strive for a perfect outcome, creating anxiety about what *might* happen. Letting go of this need for control frees up mental space, allowing you to fully experience life as it unfolds, imperfections and all.
5. **Set Boundaries for Distractions**: Social media, work obligations, and digital overload keep many people from

the present. Set specific times when you disconnect from devices, giving your mind room to exist in the current moment without distractions.

Case Study: Michael Jordan's "Flow State"

An excellent example of living in the now is *Michael Jordan* during his basketball career. Jordan was renowned not only for his skill but also for his ability to access what athletes call a "flow state," a mental space where one is completely absorbed in the moment. Jordan often described being in the zone, where time seemed to slow down, and his only focus was on the game happening in front of him.

Psychologist Mihaly Csikszentmihalyi identified this flow state as a key to achieving both high performance and deep fulfillment. Whether in sports, creative endeavors, or daily life, living in the present is the pathway to achieving mastery and inner peace.

The Path to Inner Peace

Living in the now isn't about ignoring the future or past. Instead, it's about realizing that the only moment where you have control, growth, and healing is in the present. The past can offer lessons, and the future can guide goals, but neither should consume you.

By focusing on the present, you not only manage your anxiety and stress but also connect more deeply with yourself and those around you. Every moment offers an opportunity to begin anew, to engage fully, and to find peace.

Ultimately, Law 40 is about mastering the art of presence—living fully in the now, where true healing and growth can occur.

Law 41

Find Meaning in Pain

"In some ways, suffering ceases to be suffering at the moment it finds a meaning, such as the meaning of a sacrifice."- Viktor Frankl

Pain, whether physical or emotional, often feels like an overwhelming burden, but when we view it through the lens of meaning and transformation, it becomes an engine for growth and resilience.

One way to understand the power of finding meaning in pain is through the work of psychologist Viktor Frankl, who survived the Holocaust and developed **logotherapy**, a form of existential analysis. In his seminal book *Man's Search for Meaning*, Frankl observed that the prisoners who found purpose in their suffering, whether it was through hope for the future or a sense of responsibility to something greater than themselves, were more likely to survive the brutal conditions of concentration camps. As Frankl famously said, **"When we are no longer able to change a situation, we are challenged to change ourselves."** This quote encapsulates the idea that while we may not be able to escape trauma, we can transform its meaning and impact on our lives.

Pain as a Catalyst for Growth

Psychological research has consistently shown that adversity can act as a crucible for personal growth. This phenomenon, known as **post-traumatic growth (PTG)**, refers to the positive changes that individuals often experience following significant struggles.

According to a study by Tedeschi and Calhoun (2004), approximately 90% of people who experience trauma report at least one aspect of PTG, including increased personal strength, a deeper appreciation for life, improved relationships, and a renewed sense of meaning and purpose.

Interestingly, this growth doesn't arise from the trauma itself but from how individuals respond to it. Those who engage in meaning-making, actively trying to understand how their suffering fits into a larger narrative of their life, are more likely to experience positive transformation. A 2015 study published in *Psychological Science* showed that people who engage in **cognitive reappraisal**, the process of reinterpreting an adverse event to find something meaningful within it, report lower levels of post-traumatic stress and higher levels of life satisfaction.

Finding Meaning in Painful Moments

Pain often arrives uninvited and unwanted, but it offers valuable lessons if we are willing to learn from it. To find meaning in trauma, individuals can begin by reframing their suffering. Instead of asking, "Why did this happen to me?" we can ask, "What can I learn from this experience?"

1. **Acceptance**: The first step in transforming pain is acknowledging it. Denial or avoidance only prolongs the suffering. Psychologists emphasize the importance of **radical acceptance**, a concept within Dialectical Behavior Therapy (DBT) that involves fully accepting reality as it is, without resisting or trying to change it. Only then can the healing process begin.
2. **Mindfulness**: Being present with your pain, observing it without judgment, allows you to detach from the intense emotions surrounding it. Mindfulness meditation, which has been proven to reduce anxiety and improve emotional regulation, is a powerful tool for finding calm in the midst of turmoil. Studies have shown that mindfulness can

actually rewire the brain to increase activity in areas associated with emotional regulation, such as the prefrontal cortex.

3. **Service to Others**: Often, meaning emerges through service. People who have endured significant trauma frequently find solace and purpose in helping others who are going through similar experiences. For example, individuals who have recovered from addiction often become peer counselors, supporting others in their journey to sobriety. By giving back, they transform their pain into something that benefits not only themselves but also others.

One powerful example of this is the story of **John Walsh**, who tragically lost his six-year-old son Adam to abduction and murder in 1981. Rather than succumbing to despair, Walsh dedicated his life to preventing similar tragedies. He became an advocate for missing and exploited children, co-founding the **National Center for Missing & Exploited Children** and hosting the TV show *America's Most Wanted*. Walsh's pain became a catalyst for positive change, helping countless families and ensuring that his son's death was not in vain.

Strategies to Transform Pain

To achieve this law and find meaning in trauma, one can adopt the following strategies:

- **Reflect on the Experience**: Writing about traumatic events in a journal has been shown to help individuals process their emotions. A study led by psychologist James Pennebaker found that expressive writing, where people write about their deepest thoughts and feelings related to trauma, leads to improved mental and physical health.
- **Reframe the Narrative**: Find a way to view your trauma as part of a larger narrative. Ask yourself what you have

learned from the experience, how it has shaped you, and what new opportunities it has created.

- **Seek Connection**: Building strong social connections is crucial for emotional recovery. In times of suffering, sharing your story with trusted friends, family, or a therapist can help you see the situation from different perspectives and integrate the experience in a healthy way.

- **Help Others**: Turn your pain into purpose by helping others facing similar challenges. Volunteer, mentor, or become involved in advocacy related to your experience.

Finding meaning in pain is not about erasing the scars of trauma, but about transforming those scars into sources of strength. Trauma and suffering can feel senseless and overwhelming, but by seeking out the lessons within them, we create a new narrative— one of resilience, growth, and ultimately, hope. This law encourages us to recognize that within our darkest moments lies the potential for profound personal transformation if only we are willing to engage with the pain and seek out the lessons it has to offer.

Law 42

Realign Your Priorities

"In the middle of difficulty lies opportunity." —
Albert Einstein

Trauma has a way of shattering the lens through which we view life. It forces us to pause, reflect, and often reassess the path we're on. While it may bring immense pain, it also offers an unexpected opportunity for growth by pushing us to redefine what truly matters. This realignment of priorities after trauma can catalyze personal transformation, a shift that allows us to live more authentically in line with our core values and goals.

The Transformative Power of Trauma

Research shows that many people who experience traumatic events undergo what psychologists refer to as "post-traumatic growth." This phenomenon, identified by Richard Tedeschi and Lawrence Calhoun in the 1990s, explains how some individuals emerge from their trauma not just surviving but thriving. In their studies, Tedeschi and Calhoun found that people often develop a deeper sense of purpose, a greater appreciation for life, and stronger relationships with loved ones after facing adversity.

Take the case of Jane McGonigal, a video game designer who, after suffering a traumatic brain injury, found herself in a deep depression. Her once busy and fulfilling life came to a screeching halt, leaving her physically debilitated and mentally shattered. However, instead of succumbing to her suffering, McGonigal used her experience as fuel to reassess what truly mattered to her. She discovered a passion for helping others heal through play and created a game called "SuperBetter," designed to help people recover from trauma. Her personal journey through trauma reshaped her priorities, transforming her career and ultimately allowing her to help millions of others realign their own lives.

The Science of Reassessing Priorities

When trauma strikes, the brain undergoes significant changes, particularly in the areas responsible for emotion, memory, and decision-making. Neuroplasticity, the brain's ability to reorganize itself by forming new neural connections, is at the heart of this transformation. Studies show that individuals who practice mindfulness, reflection, and intentional goal-setting after trauma can strengthen the brain's pathways for resilience and emotional regulation. These practices also allow the brain to shed unhealthy habits and thought patterns, replacing them with ones more aligned with personal growth and well-being.

A well-known study conducted by researchers at the University of North Carolina examined how mindfulness and intentional reflection can help trauma survivors realign their lives. The study found that individuals who engaged in these practices reported significantly higher levels of life satisfaction, greater clarity on personal values, and a renewed sense of purpose compared to those who did not engage in such practices. The process of pausing and reassessing after trauma can serve as a reset button, enabling us to redefine our priorities and pursue goals that align with our true selves.

Realigning After Trauma: A Process of Rediscovery

Realigning your priorities after trauma involves a process of rediscovery. This begins with acceptance—acknowledging the trauma and its impact on your life without letting it define your future. From there, intentional reflection allows you to assess the areas of your life that no longer serve you. Whether it's a toxic relationship, an unfulfilling career, or a personal belief system that no longer aligns with your values, trauma can provide the clarity needed to make the hard choices for a more authentic life.

One example of this process is found in the story of Andre Agassi, the former tennis champion. Agassi was at the top of his career, but despite his success, he admitted that he hated tennis. His rise to fame was driven by external expectations and a desire to please others, but an injury that nearly ended his career forced him to reevaluate. In his autobiography *Open*, Agassi speaks about how the trauma of his injury and personal struggles led him to rediscover his passion—not for tennis, but for philanthropy. He went on to establish the Andre Agassi Foundation for Education, which builds schools for underprivileged children. Trauma realigned his priorities, pushing him toward a more purpose-driven life.

The Roadmap to Realignment: Strategies for Reassessing Your Priorities

Achieving Law 42, realigning your priorities after trauma, is not an instantaneous process—it requires intentional effort. Below are steps that can guide you through this transformative journey:

1. **Self-Reflection:** Take time to ask yourself what truly matters. Trauma often strips away the distractions and forces you to confront the essential aspects of life—what you value, what brings you joy, and what fulfills you. Journaling, meditation, or simply spending time in nature can help facilitate this reflection.
2. **Set New Goals:** Trauma changes you, and your goals should reflect this new reality. What do you want to achieve moving forward? Perhaps it's not the high-powered career you once pursued, but instead, a desire to help others or spend more time with family. Aligning your

goals with your core values will provide a sense of direction.

3. **Embrace Growth:** As Viktor Frankl, a Holocaust survivor and renowned psychiatrist, once said, "When we are no longer able to change a situation, we are challenged to change ourselves." View your trauma as an opportunity for growth, allowing it to guide you toward a more meaningful existence. Growth may come from seeking therapy, taking on new challenges, or engaging in volunteer work— whatever fosters your personal evolution.

4. **Seek Support:** Realigning your priorities doesn't have to be a solo journey. Surround yourself with a support system that encourages and uplifts you. Whether through close friends, family, or professional support groups, community is crucial to the healing process. Studies show that trauma survivors who have strong social connections report higher levels of well-being and resilience.

5. **Let Go of What No Longer Serves You:** Trauma teaches you the importance of shedding the unnecessary— whether it's unhealthy relationships, old habits, or limiting beliefs. As you realign your priorities, give yourself permission to let go of the things that no longer contribute to your growth and happiness.

Moving Forward with Purpose

Ultimately, trauma can act as a powerful force of redirection. While it may feel like everything is falling apart, it also presents an opportunity to rebuild. By realigning your priorities in the aftermath of trauma, you are able to live more authentically, in alignment with your core values and purpose. Through reflection, goal-setting, and embracing growth, you transform trauma into a source of strength, using it to guide you toward what truly matters.

Trauma reshapes you, but it does not have to break you. Instead, let it guide you—just as it has for countless individuals—toward a life that is more fulfilling, intentional, and aligned with your deepest values.

Law 43

Seek Inner Peace

"Peace comes from within. Do not seek it without."
- Buddha

Inner peace is not something that happens by chance—it's a state of mind cultivated through conscious practice, a calm that can withstand life's storms. While the world around us may be in chaos, we can foster an inner sanctuary through deliberate habits and self-awareness. **Inner peace is not the absence of conflict; it is the ability to maintain calm amidst challenges.** To achieve this peace, you must learn to control your reactions and strengthen your mental fortitude. The law of **"Seek Inner Peace"** invites us to consciously cultivate practices that nurture this peace within us, making us more resilient to external forces.

Seeking inner peace is about fostering a mindset that remains calm and balanced despite life's inevitable challenges. **One key to achieving this peace is through mindfulness and meditation**, both of which have been extensively studied for their profound impact on mental and emotional well-being. In a study published in *JAMA Internal Medicine*, researchers found that individuals who practiced mindfulness-based stress reduction experienced significant reductions in anxiety, depression, and stress. These practices help you center yourself, allowing you to remain focused on the present moment rather than getting lost in past regrets or future anxieties.

Resilience through Meditation

Meditation is not just a spiritual practice but a scientifically supported tool for calming the mind and body. A study by Harvard neuroscientist Sara Lazar showed that meditation could physically alter the brain. MRI scans of meditators revealed thickening in the prefrontal cortex, which is responsible for higher-order thinking and emotional regulation. This evidence supports the idea that with regular practice, meditation can strengthen your ability to manage emotions, helping you maintain inner peace in stressful situations.

Inner Peace Amidst Chaos: Learning from Examples

Inner peace can be maintained even in the midst of external chaos, as demonstrated by the story of **Wangari Maathai**, the Nobel laureate who founded the Green Belt Movement in Kenya. Despite facing political oppression, threats to her life, and imprisonment, Maathai remained centered in her mission. She stated, *"It's the little things citizens do. That's what will make the difference. My little thing is planting trees."* Her ability to maintain focus on her goal—planting millions of trees across Africa—demonstrates how inner peace comes from having a clear purpose and aligning your actions with that purpose.

Likewise, the stoic philosopher **Marcus Aurelius** once said, *"You have power over your mind, not outside events. Realize this, and you will find strength."* His words echo the essence of this law, emphasizing that true peace is found in controlling our inner reactions, not the external world.

Techniques to Cultivate Inner Peace

1. **Mindfulness and Meditation:** These practices help in calming the mind, bringing awareness to the present moment, and fostering a deep sense of connection with oneself. Harvard Medical School research has shown that mindfulness reduces levels of the stress hormone cortisol, creating a more relaxed state.

2. **Journaling:** Reflecting on your thoughts and emotions through journaling can help declutter the mind. Writing down your worries allows you to confront and process them, rather than letting them swirl around in your head.

3. **Gratitude Practice:** Consistently practicing gratitude can transform your mindset and shift your focus from what's lacking to what's abundant in your life. Studies have shown that people who regularly express gratitude are generally happier and experience lower levels of stress.

4. **Exercise and Physical Activity:** Physical movement is crucial for emotional well-being. Studies have shown that regular exercise releases endorphins, the body's natural stress relievers, which help to keep you emotionally balanced and grounded.

The Science of Inner Peace

Peace within is not an abstract concept, but a real physiological state. Research conducted at the University of Wisconsin-Madison's Center for Healthy Minds revealed that practicing mindfulness increases activity in the left prefrontal cortex—the part of the brain associated with happiness and calm. It also reduces activity in the amygdala, the brain's fear center, indicating that inner peace can actually rewire the brain for long-term emotional resilience.

How to Achieve Law 43: Seek Inner Peace

To truly master the art of inner peace, you must integrate daily practices that foster it. Consider adopting these habits:

1. **Start Each Day with Meditation:** Even 5-10 minutes of meditation can set a peaceful tone for the day ahead. Focus on your breath, clear your mind, and let go of any lingering stress.

2. **Engage in a Daily Gratitude Practice:** Write down three things you're grateful for each day. This simple act can help shift your mindset towards positivity and calm.

3. **Limit Exposure to Negative Energy:** Whether it's toxic relationships or media that triggers anxiety, be mindful of what and who you allow into your mental space. Create boundaries to protect your peace.

4. **Connect with Nature:** Spending time outdoors has been shown to reduce stress and promote feelings of calm and connection. Even a short walk in a park can rejuvenate your mental state.

Inner peace is not a one-time achievement, but a lifelong practice. Like a garden, it must be nurtured regularly, through mindfulness, intentional practices, and a commitment to self-care. **In the words of Lao Tzu**, *"If you are depressed, you are living in the past. If you are anxious, you are living in the future. If you are at peace, you are living in the present."* The key to achieving Law 43 is recognizing that peace is cultivated from within, not found in the absence of problems. By focusing on the present and using life's challenges as opportunities for growth, you can build a fortress of calm within yourself that no external circumstance can shake.

Law 44

Be Consistent in Your Practices

It's not what we do once in a while that shapes our lives, but what we do consistently."
— *Tony Robbins*

Be Consistent in Your Practices underscores the transformative power of consistent, deliberate effort in achieving lasting healing and growth. Healing, whether from trauma, mental stress, or emotional pain, is not a one-time event but a continual process that requires commitment and persistence. This law is anchored in the simple truth that consistency is the key to achieving profound, sustainable change.

In many aspects of life, consistency is the cornerstone of success, and healing is no different. The idea of gradual but steady progress is central to a growing body of research that underscores how the brain and body adapt to repeated, intentional effort. According to studies in **neuroplasticity**, the brain changes its structure and function in response to consistent practice and experiences. This process is vital for healing from trauma or emotional wounds, as it allows new neural pathways to form, slowly replacing the old, maladaptive responses with healthier ones.

One famous study on trauma and recovery, the **Adverse Childhood Experiences (ACE) study**, highlights the long-term impacts of trauma on health, behavior, and relationships. However, it also shows that with consistent support, therapy, and mindfulness practices, even individuals with high ACE scores can recover and lead fulfilling lives. Consistent practices such as meditation, therapy, physical exercise, and positive relationships help restore the brain's ability to regulate emotions, reduce anxiety, and foster resilience.

The Power of Consistency in Healing Practices

Consistency is a transformative force, yet it's often underestimated in its simplicity. Many of the most significant breakthroughs in trauma recovery and mental health have been grounded in consistent practice. Take **Cognitive Behavioral Therapy (CBT)** as an example. This widely used therapeutic approach relies heavily on regular, repeated efforts to reshape thought patterns and behaviors. Studies have shown that patients who engage in consistent CBT sessions over time experience more significant reductions in anxiety and depression compared to those who attend therapy sporadically.

The idea is simple: small, repeated actions compound over time, leading to larger changes in mood, behavior, and overall well-being. Imagine each therapy session, each mindful meditation, or each self-care activity as a single drop of water. Alone, it might seem insignificant, but over time, these drops fill a container of healing and resilience. This is the power of consistency.

Historical Instances of Consistent Practice Leading to Healing

Consider the story of **Louisa May Alcott**, the famous author of *Little Women*. Throughout her life, Alcott faced numerous physical and emotional challenges, including illness and familial financial instability. Yet, she developed a disciplined writing practice, consistently working on her craft as a form of both expression and healing. Her ability to create beauty out of adversity was not born out of sudden inspiration but through the steady, persistent act of writing, day after day. Alcott's consistency not only allowed her to produce one of America's most beloved novels but also provided her with a way to process and rise above her personal struggles.

Similarly, **Winston Churchill**, known for his leadership during World War II, struggled with depression—what he called his "black dog." Churchill did not conquer his depression through a single, sweeping action but through the consistent application of practices that helped him cope. From maintaining a regular routine to engaging in creative outlets like painting and writing, Churchill's steady efforts enabled him to manage his mental health even in the face of extraordinary stress.

How to Achieve Law 44: The Path of Consistency

Achieving consistency in healing practices requires both intention and discipline. Here are several steps to help build this practice into your daily life:

1. **Start Small**: Begin with manageable actions that you can repeat daily. Whether it's setting aside five minutes for mindfulness or scheduling weekly therapy sessions, starting small allows you to build momentum.
2. **Create a Routine**: Healing requires structure. Establish a routine that incorporates consistent healing practices, whether it's journaling, mindfulness meditation, physical exercise, or time spent in nature. A study published in the journal *Mindfulness* found that individuals who maintained a regular mindfulness practice had greater emotional regulation and decreased stress levels than those with irregular practices.
3. **Set Clear Intentions**: Define what you're trying to heal or change. Is it your anxiety, your response to trauma, or a sense of disconnectedness? Having a clear goal helps you stay focused on your practice and understand the purpose behind your consistency.
4. **Track Your Progress**: Research from **Harvard Business School** on habit formation shows that tracking your progress leads to higher rates of success. By keeping a journal of your daily practices and noting changes, you'll

not only remain motivated but also recognize the cumulative impact of your efforts.

5. **Lean on Support**: Surround yourself with a support system that encourages your healing journey. Whether it's friends, a therapist, or an online community, consistent encouragement and accountability can significantly bolster your efforts.

6. **Practice Self-Compassion**: Healing is not linear, and there will be days when you feel like you've made little progress. Be kind to yourself and recognize that consistency isn't about perfection—it's about showing up, even on difficult days.

Research and Statistics: Consistency Matters

A **meta-analysis published in _JAMA Psychiatry_** examined the effects of consistent psychotherapy sessions on patients with PTSD. The study found that individuals who attended therapy regularly experienced a 68% greater reduction in symptoms compared to those who attended sporadically. The power of consistency was clear: small, regular engagements with therapy led to meaningful, lasting improvements.

In another study on the **effects of meditation**, researchers found that participants who meditated daily for eight weeks had a significant decrease in stress levels, improved focus, and increased feelings of well-being compared to those who meditated intermittently. Regular mindfulness practice has been linked to reduced anxiety, lower cortisol levels (the body's stress hormone), and improved emotional resilience.

The Lasting Impact of Consistent Healing Practices

Consistent action leads to lasting transformation. Whether it's the small act of checking in with yourself daily or the ongoing commitment to therapy or mindfulness, consistency is the bridge between where you are now and where you want to be. By showing up for yourself regularly, you harness the power to create deeper recovery, resilience, and emotional growth.

Trauma and emotional pain can leave us feeling like healing is impossible, but consistency allows us to take small steps forward, day by day until the cumulative impact leads to profound change. Like steel forged in fire, our emotional and mental resilience is built over time, through the consistent application of effort, care, and intention.

In the end, the key to mastering Law 44 is the same as mastering anything of value in life: you must show up, regularly and with intention, for your own healing journey. The process is long, but with each consistent step, you move closer to becoming the best version of yourself.

Victor O. Carl

Law 45

Honor Your Progress

"It does not matter how slowly you go as long as you do not stop."– Confucius

Honor Your Progress reminds us that growth is a journey, not a single event. Every small step forward, every challenge you overcome, is a sign of progress worth recognizing. This law highlights the importance of reflecting on how far you've come, which not only reinforces resilience but also motivates you to continue moving forward.

In our fast-paced world, it is easy to get caught up in the pursuit of bigger goals and forget to acknowledge the progress we have made along the way. Recognizing your achievements, no matter how small, is a crucial step in building mental strength. According to research published by Teresa Amabile of Harvard Business School, the **"progress principle"** suggests that even incremental steps toward a goal can have a profound impact on an individual's emotional state and motivation. People who track and celebrate their progress are more likely to be engaged, motivated, and ultimately successful in their endeavors.

Progress as Motivation

The act of reflecting on and honoring your progress is not just about patting yourself on the back; it's about creating momentum. The **Zeigarnik effect**, a psychological phenomenon that explains why people tend to remember unfinished tasks more vividly than completed ones, shows that the brain is wired to focus on what remains to be done rather than what has already been

231

accomplished. But when we make a conscious effort to celebrate our achievements, we create positive reinforcement loops that increase our overall motivation.

For example, consider the experience of **James Dyson**, the British inventor who took more than 5,000 prototypes before perfecting his revolutionary vacuum cleaner. Every failed prototype could have been seen as a step backward, but Dyson chose to focus on what he was learning with each iteration. Honoring his progress gave him the resilience to continue, eventually leading to massive commercial success and a lasting impact on the home appliance industry. Dyson's story is a powerful illustration of how acknowledging progress can fuel resilience and persistence.

The Psychological Benefits of Celebrating Small Wins

Psychologically, celebrating small wins has a profound impact on well-being. According to a study published in the journal **Emotion**, positive emotions experienced during moments of progress contribute to greater life satisfaction, increased motivation, and enhanced performance. These moments of recognition encourage individuals to savor their achievements, reinforcing the idea that growth is ongoing and multifaceted.

In fact, research shows that people who journal about their progress and reflect on positive steps forward often experience a significant increase in self-efficacy—the belief in one's ability to succeed. This self-efficacy is a critical component of **resilience**, the mental muscle that allows individuals to bounce back from adversity. When we take the time to honor our progress, we strengthen our belief in ourselves, creating a foundation for future success.

Historical Examples of Progress

History is filled with examples of individuals who understood the power of honoring progress. **Thomas Edison**, the inventor of the lightbulb, famously noted, *"I have not failed. I've just found 10,000 ways that won't work."* Edison's ability to honor his learning progress rather than dwell on failure enabled him to persist through countless setbacks. His acknowledgment of every experiment as a step forward in his journey exemplifies the essence of Law 45.

Another example can be found in the life of **J.K. Rowling**, the author of the Harry Potter series. Before achieving global success, Rowling faced numerous rejections from publishers, financial struggles, and personal setbacks. But instead of focusing on her failures, she kept writing, continually celebrating the progress she made in her storytelling. Her resilience and recognition of incremental progress led her to create one of the most beloved literary franchises in history.

Practical Steps to Honor Your Progress

Honoring your progress doesn't have to be a grand gesture; it can be done through simple, intentional actions. Here are practical steps to help you incorporate this law into your daily life:

1. **Journaling**: At the end of each day, take a few minutes to reflect on what you've accomplished, no matter how small. Writing it down reinforces your achievements and gives you a tangible record of your growth.
2. **Visualizing Growth**: Create a visual progress chart where you track your steps toward a goal. This could be as simple as marking off a calendar or using an app that lets you log your milestones.
3. **Celebrate Small Wins**: Don't wait for the final goal to reward yourself. Celebrate small wins by treating yourself to something special—whether that's a moment of rest, a walk, or something you enjoy.
4. **Reflect Regularly**: Schedule time to reflect on your larger progress at key milestones, such as the end of a month or

after completing a significant task. Acknowledge what you've learned and how far you've come.

5. **Positive Affirmation**: Remind yourself daily of your strengths and abilities. Positive self-talk can be a powerful tool for building confidence and reinforcing a sense of accomplishment.

By implementing these practices, you create a habit of honoring your growth. This not only fuels motivation but also builds a strong sense of resilience, allowing you to face future challenges with confidence and strength.

Law 45: Honor Your Progress teaches that every forward movement is a reason to celebrate, as it strengthens your resolve and builds a foundation for future success. Honoring your progress allows you to look back at the obstacles you've overcome, turning them into stepping stones rather than roadblocks. As you continue on your journey, remember that growth is not always linear, but each step forward, no matter how small, brings you closer to your goals.

Law 46

Rediscover Who You Are

"I am not what happened to me, I am what I choose to become." – Carl Jung

"Trauma can obscure, but it can also reveal your true self." At its core, trauma often strips away the layers of identity, plunging us into confusion and darkness. However, it also presents an opportunity to rebuild and rediscover a more authentic version of ourselves. By actively reconnecting with our identity, passions, and what makes us unique, we can transcend the pain of the past and step into a new era of self-awareness and personal growth.

When we experience trauma, our sense of self can become fragmented, leading to feelings of alienation and loss. Studies have shown that trauma can have long-lasting effects on our identity, often masking who we are at our core. For example, research on PTSD demonstrates how traumatic experiences can result in a shift in personality, values, and relationships. Individuals may find themselves detached from their former passions or even their very sense of purpose. Yet, amid the chaos, the true self often remains—waiting to be rediscovered.

To fully grasp this concept, let's look at historical evidence. The concept of post-traumatic growth (PTG) provides a framework for understanding how individuals can thrive after experiencing adversity. Developed by psychologists Richard Tedeschi and Lawrence Calhoun in the 1990s, PTG suggests that many individuals not only recover from trauma but also find a greater sense of meaning, purpose, and personal strength afterward. This paradigm shift in psychology emphasizes that the path to healing is not just about survival, but about flourishing and reconnecting with one's inner self.

Rediscovery Through Reflection: The Journey Inward

Reconnecting with your true self is a journey that requires reflection, self-awareness, and emotional honesty. According to a study published in the JOURNAL OF TRAUMATIC STRESS, practices like mindfulness, journaling, and self-reflection are critical tools for individuals to understand how trauma has impacted their sense of self. Taking time to introspect allows you to sift through the emotional debris and rediscover the passions, values, and beliefs that define you.

For instance, during the aftermath of the 9/11 attacks, many survivors reported experiencing a newfound clarity about what mattered most in their lives. While the trauma was devastating, it also forced individuals to reflect on their relationships, values, and goals. Many found a renewed sense of purpose and a stronger connection to their inner selves after coming to terms with the experience.

Breaking Through the Trauma: Techniques for Rediscovery

To achieve Law 46—Rediscover Who You Are—certain techniques can help you peel back the layers of trauma and reengage with your authentic self:

1. **Mindfulness and Meditation:**

Numerous studies, including research from the AMERICAN PSYCHOLOGICAL ASSOCIATION, have shown that mindfulness meditation not only reduces anxiety but also enhances self-awareness. By practicing mindfulness, individuals can quiet the mental noise caused by trauma and reconnect with the deeper layers of their identity. Meditation fosters a compassionate relationship with oneself, which is critical for rediscovery.

2. **Creative Expression:**

Artistic expression—whether through writing, painting, or music—allows for the release of pent-up emotions. Research from the HARVARD MEDICAL SCHOOL suggests that creative activities promote healing by helping individuals articulate the emotions that they may not be able to put into words. Through creativity, we access parts of our identity that have been buried by trauma.

3. **Engaging in New Experiences:**

Trauma can often lead to avoidance behaviors, where individuals retreat from the world. However, by stepping into new experiences—whether through travel, learning a new skill, or forming new relationships—individuals can rediscover forgotten aspects of themselves. Positive psychology research has shown that engaging in novel experiences helps reignite the joy and passion often lost in the shadow of trauma.

4. **Therapeutic Techniques:**

   Professional support is essential for many in the process of rediscovery. Therapy models such as Internal Family Systems (IFS) focus on healing the internal dialogue within oneself, helping individuals rediscover their "true self" by addressing the parts of them that were wounded in the trauma. Cognitive Behavioral Therapy (CBT) and Eye Movement Desensitization and Reprocessing (EMDR) are also effective in bringing clarity to the post-trauma experience, helping individuals step out of the confusion of their past and into the present.

Embracing Your True Self: The Power of Acceptance

An essential aspect of rediscovering who you are involves accepting your new reality. Trauma changes us, often irreversibly. However, as philosopher Friedrich Nietzsche once said, **"That which does not kill us makes us stronger."** Rather than seeing the self before trauma as the "true" self, one must embrace the self that has emerged from the wreckage. This new version of yourself carries the wisdom, resilience, and emotional depth that only adversity can teach.

Take the story of Maya Angelou. Although she endured a traumatic childhood—being raped at the age of 8 and subsequently going mute for five years—she ultimately found her voice as one of the most profound literary figures in American history. Angelou's trauma may have obscured her voice for a time, but her journey of rediscovery allowed her to reclaim her identity and use her experiences to shape her future contributions to literature and civil rights.

Rediscovering who you are after trauma is not about inventing a new self—it's about reclaiming the self that was always there, underneath the pain. Trauma may obscure your sense of identity, but it does not erase it. With the right tools—reflection, mindfulness, creativity, and support—you can peel back the layers of trauma and reconnect with the essence of who you are, stronger and more resilient than before.

Law 47

Embrace the Journey

"It is good to have an end to journey toward; but it is the journey that matters, in the end."
— *Ursula K. Le Guin*

"Healing is a path, not a destination; it is a continuous journey filled with growth, setbacks, and transformation." This law emphasizes the importance of embracing the process of healing rather than fixating on an endpoint. In our fast-paced, outcome-driven world, we often seek quick solutions and final resolutions. But true healing, especially from trauma and deep emotional wounds, is not something that can be achieved overnight or through a singular breakthrough—it is a lifelong process of learning, self-discovery, and adaptation.

The Journey of Healing: A Gradual Unfolding

Understanding that healing is a journey requires a mindset shift. It involves letting go of the notion that there is a final point of "being healed." Instead, it recognizes that healing is cyclical, with its own ups and downs. Psychologists refer to this process as "nonlinear recovery." Research from the AMERICAN PSYCHOLOGICAL ASSOCIATION shows that trauma recovery does not follow a straight line; individuals often experience periods of progress followed by setbacks. This is natural and part of the journey.

One well-known example of this idea comes from the work of Dr. Judith Herman, a pioneer in the field of trauma recovery. Her seminal book TRAUMA AND RECOVERY outlines the stages of healing: establishing safety, remembrance and mourning, and reconnection with ordinary life. These stages are not rigid steps but rather overlapping and recurrent experiences. As Herman explains, survivors may revisit earlier stages multiple times, emphasizing that healing is an ongoing, evolving process.

Embracing the Process: Finding Meaning in Every Step

One of the most powerful ways to embrace the journey is to find meaning in every step—whether that step is one of progress or one of challenge. Viktor Frankl, a Holocaust survivor and the founder of logotherapy highlighted the significance of finding purpose in suffering. In his book MAN'S SEARCH FOR MEANING, he stated, **"In some ways, suffering ceases to be suffering at the moment it finds a meaning, such as the meaning of a sacrifice."** This approach to healing transforms the way we view setbacks. Instead of seeing them as failures, we can see them as opportunities for growth and understanding.

Navigating Setbacks with Compassion

Setbacks are an inevitable part of any healing journey. Yet, many people feel frustrated when they encounter obstacles or experience a resurgence of old wounds. Psychological research on self-compassion, led by Dr. Kristin Neff, demonstrates that individuals who approach themselves with kindness during difficult moments are more likely to experience emotional resilience. Self-compassion involves treating yourself with the same understanding and patience that you would offer a friend who is struggling. Studies show that practicing self-compassion not only improves emotional well-being but also accelerates recovery from trauma by reducing feelings of shame and self-blame.

Take, for example, the life of Maya Angelou (without referring to her as the focus of the story). In her memoirs, Angelou shares how she repeatedly faced personal challenges, yet she continued to rebuild her life after each setback. Her life illustrates how healing is not linear but rather a journey that requires perseverance, self-reflection, and acceptance of each stage.

Cultural and Historical Examples of Embracing the Journey

Throughout history, cultures have recognized that healing is an evolving process. The traditional Japanese concept of WABI-SABI captures this beautifully. WABI-SABI embraces the beauty in imperfection, seeing the incomplete or broken as part of life's natural flow. A famous practice rooted in this philosophy is KINTSUGI—the art of repairing broken pottery with gold. Rather than hiding the cracks, KINTSUGI highlights them, celebrating the object's history and making it more beautiful in its imperfection. This serves as a metaphor for the healing journey: rather than trying to return to a pre-trauma state, we learn to integrate our scars, recognizing that they are part of our unique story.

The Maasai people of East Africa have a similar cultural tradition. Warriors who have been wounded in battle are given time to heal, not just physically but emotionally, in a process that includes communal rituals and songs. These rituals emphasize that the warrior's wounds are part of the collective journey, and their recovery is seen as a process that strengthens the entire community.

How to Achieve Law 47: Practical Strategies

1. **Shift Your Focus from Destination to Process:**

   Many people set rigid goals for their healing journey, such as "I need to feel better in six months." This focus on outcomes can lead to disappointment. Instead, shift your mindset to focus on the process. Celebrate small wins, whether it's a day without anxiety, a moment of joy, or simply recognizing a negative thought without reacting to it.

2. **Accept the Ebb and Flow of Healing:**

   Healing is not a constant upward trajectory. Dr. Bessel van der Kolk, author of THE BODY KEEPS THE SCORE, explains that recovery from trauma often involves periods where the body and mind return to old patterns. Recognizing that these setbacks are normal can help reduce frustration and despair. Rather than seeing them as failures, view them as part of the natural rhythm of recovery.

3. **Practice Self-Compassion:**

   As Dr. Kristin Neff's research shows, self-compassion is a powerful tool for healing. When you experience a setback, offer yourself words of encouragement rather than criticism. Remind yourself that healing is difficult and that you are doing the best you can in each moment.

4. **Find Joy in the Small Moments:**

Healing doesn't just happen in therapy sessions or during intense periods of self-reflection. It happens in the quiet, everyday moments of life. As you go through your healing journey, find joy in the small things—a walk in nature, a good meal, a conversation with a friend. These moments help build emotional resilience and remind you that life is not just about overcoming pain; it's also about experiencing beauty.

5. **Seek Out Supportive Communities:**

Healing is rarely achieved in isolation. In fact, studies show that individuals who have a strong support system recover more quickly from trauma. The key is to find communities that understand and support your healing journey. Whether it's a group of friends, a therapy group, or even an online community, having others who walk alongside you can make the journey less lonely.

Conclusion: The Journey Is the Destination

In embracing Law 47—EMBRACE THE JOURNEY—you realize that healing is not about reaching an endpoint. It is about navigating the twists and turns with patience, grace, and self-compassion. Each step forward, each setback, and each moment of reflection is an opportunity for growth. The journey itself becomes the destination as you learn to accept the process as part of your larger personal evolution.

As the ancient philosopher Lao Tzu once said, **"A journey of a thousand miles begins with a single step."** The secret is not in how quickly you reach the end but in how fully you embrace every step along the way.

Law 48

Believe in Your Power

"The most common way people give up their power is by thinking they don't have any."
— *Alice Walker*

You are stronger than you know; resilience is your birthright. The human spirit has an innate capacity for endurance, recovery, and growth—an inner well of strength waiting to be tapped. Often, we underestimate our ability to overcome life's challenges, yet history and science have shown time and again that individuals possess an extraordinary power to heal, adapt, and thrive, even in the face of overwhelming adversity. Believing in your own resilience is not just an abstract concept, it is a mindset backed by research and lived experiences across time. This law calls on you to embrace that belief and understand that your ability to heal and succeed is greater than you realize.

Breaking Old Agreements: Understanding Personal Freedom and Strength

We often speak of freedom—whether it's political freedom, personal freedom, or emotional freedom. But true freedom is much more profound; it is the freedom to be who we *really* are, unshackled by external expectations, social conditioning, or internal limitations. Many of us live in invisible prisons constructed by past experiences, old agreements, or limiting beliefs. These self-imposed barriers make us doubt our own potential. As psychologist Viktor Frankl observed during his time in Nazi concentration camps, "Everything can be taken from a man but one thing: the last of the human freedoms—to choose one's attitude in any given set of circumstances, to choose one's own way." This quote reminds us that no matter the situation, we have the power to reclaim our freedom and control our inner world.

To understand how to break free from these mental and emotional barriers, consider the example of *placebo effects* in medicine. Numerous studies have demonstrated that when patients believe they are receiving effective treatment, even when they are given a sugar pill, they often experience real improvements in their condition. This phenomenon is so well-documented that it has been studied in multiple medical trials over the years, including those involving chronic pain, depression, and anxiety. It serves as a reminder that belief alone has immense power to change both the mind and the body, indicating the deep connection between resilience and our own convictions.

Understanding Your Inner Strength: The Science of Resilience

One of the most remarkable findings in modern psychology is the understanding of **resilience**—the ability to bounce back from adversity. In the aftermath of disasters, wars, or traumatic experiences, a significant number of people not only survive but thrive. Psychologist George A. Bonanno coined the term *"resilience trajectory"* to describe this process, showing that resilience isn't just about returning to a pre-crisis state but often involves growth beyond it. His studies of survivors of trauma revealed that upwards of 50% of people demonstrate natural resilience, while others can learn to develop it.

The question, then, is how do we nurture this innate strength? The answer lies in shifting the narratives we tell ourselves, much like breaking old agreements. In **Carol Dweck's research on "growth mindset,"** individuals who believe they can improve through effort and learning are far more likely to persevere through challenges and achieve success. They are not limited by failure; instead, they view it as a part of the journey towards growth. This kind of mindset shift empowers individuals to confront obstacles head-on, believing that their internal capacity can rise to meet the demands of any challenge.

The Power of Belief: Historical Examples of Strength

History is replete with stories of individuals and communities who faced insurmountable odds and, through sheer inner strength and belief, not only survived but changed the world. Consider the story of **Hiroo Onoda**, a Japanese soldier who continued to fight World War II for nearly three decades after it had officially ended. Refusing to believe the war was over, Onoda remained in the jungles of the Philippines, driven by an unwavering sense of duty. His story exemplifies the power of belief in one's own mission and strength, even in the most extreme circumstances.

Or take the case of **Bethany Hamilton**, the surfer who lost her arm in a shark attack at the age of 13. Rather than giving up, she not only returned to surfing but became a professional, competing in major championships. Her story of resilience isn't just about physical recovery—it's about mental fortitude, self-belief, and the will to pursue her passion despite a life-altering setback.

In both cases, these individuals believed in their own capacity to overcome adversity, even when the world told them otherwise. Their success was rooted in an unwavering conviction that their inner strength would carry them through. This same strength lies within all of us.

How to Achieve the 48th Law: Belief in Your Power

Achieving this 48th law of mental power—*believing in your own strength*—requires several key steps that are rooted in both mindset and practice:

1. **Challenge Limiting Beliefs**: Recognize and confront the agreements and beliefs that hold you back. Ask yourself: Are

these beliefs truly serving you, or are they relics of past conditioning? Just as **Toltec wisdom** teaches, we must identify and dismantle the "parasite" in our minds—the judge and the victim—that thrives on our emotional wounds. Begin by replacing fear-based beliefs with empowering ones, and slowly, you will reclaim your power.

2. **Practice Resilience**: Like any skill, resilience grows with practice. Studies have shown that resilience can be nurtured through *positive coping mechanisms* such as mindfulness, social support, and purposeful action. Engaging in *mindfulness-based stress reduction* (MBSR) has been found to reduce the psychological impact of stress, trauma, and adversity. These techniques help you stay grounded and focused, allowing you to face challenges with calm and clarity.

3. **Surround Yourself with Empowerment**: The people around you have a significant impact on your mindset. Studies have revealed that **social connections** are one of the strongest predictors of resilience. In times of struggle, humans instinctively reach out to others for support, and those who cultivate strong, positive relationships often recover faster from adversity. Align yourself with individuals and communities who lift you up and reinforce your belief in your own strength.

4. **Celebrate Small Wins**: Every time you confront a fear or overcome an obstacle, no matter how small, you strengthen your belief in yourself. Psychologist **Charles Duhigg** explains in his book *The Power of Habit* that small victories are crucial in building momentum. As you achieve these wins, your sense of control and belief in your abilities will grow, empowering you to tackle bigger challenges.

Believing in your power is not just a platitude—it is a call to action. It is the recognition that resilience is a birthright, one that is cultivated through awareness, effort, and the breaking of old agreements. You have the strength within you to overcome whatever life throws your way, just as countless others have before you. The path to personal power lies in trusting yourself, embracing your innate resilience, and harnessing the extraordinary capacity of the human spirit to thrive.

CONCLUSION

As we reach the end of this exploration into the 48 Laws of Mental Power, it's important to remember that the journey doesn't end here. The path to mental resilience is a lifelong endeavor, one that requires constant practice, self-reflection, and a willingness to embrace both the challenges and the triumphs that life throws our way.

Throughout this book, we've delved into the depths of the human psyche, exploring the intricate workings of the mind and the profound impact of trauma, adversity, and resilience. We've learned from the wisdom of ancient philosophers, the insights of modern psychologists, and the inspiring stories of individuals who have overcome seemingly insurmountable obstacles.

The 48 Laws of Mental Power are not just abstract concepts; they are practical tools that can be applied to your daily life. By incorporating these laws into your mindset and actions, you can cultivate a mental fortitude that empowers you to navigate life's complexities with grace, strength, and unwavering resolve.

Remember, the journey to mental power is not about achieving perfection; it's about progress. It's about recognizing your strengths, acknowledging your vulnerabilities, and embracing the continuous process of growth and transformation.

As you continue on this path, remember that you are not alone. You are part of a vast community of individuals who are also striving to cultivate mental resilience and live more fulfilling lives. Reach out to others, share your experiences, and support each other on this journey.

The world needs your strength, your compassion, and your unique perspective. By embracing the 48 Laws of Mental Power, you are not only transforming your own life but also contributing to a more resilient and empowered world.

The journey continues. Embrace it, learn from it, and let it shape you into the best version of yourself.

About the Author

Victor O. Carl is the pen name of a visionary researcher and author whose mission is to empower individuals to unlock their full potential. With a background rooted in extensive research and a passion for personal growth, Carl has authored several transformative books.

His first book, *The 48 Laws of Mental Power*, takes readers deep into the unseen forces driving human behavior, unlocking strategies to sharpen the mind and fortify inner resilience. Carl continued his quest for self-mastery in *The 48 Laws of Habit Mastery*, delivering timeless methods to transform routines and habits into tools of success. With *The 48 Laws of Money*, Carl demystifies the secrets of wealth-building, bridging psychology and financial wisdom, while *The 48 Laws of Peace* offers readers a path to inner tranquility in an increasingly chaotic world.

Carl's books are not just guides but manuals for survival in a world designed to overwhelm the individual. Drawing from his profound experiences and deep research, he challenges readers to transcend the limitations imposed by society and their own conditioning. His work is crafted for those who are ready to break free, master themselves, and achieve lasting transformation. You can Visit his website below For Updates.

www.48lol.com

Acknowledgments

I am deeply grateful to my family, especially my wife and kids (Videl, Vishal, and Valen), and to my friends for their unwavering support and belief in my vision. To the mentors and thinkers whose ideas shaped these works—thank you for your invaluable guidance.

A heartfelt thanks to my readers, whose curiosity and dedication to personal growth inspire me to continue writing. These books are for all who seek mastery over their minds, habits, and lives.

Thank you for being part of this journey.